MIND
BODY
F.I.T. *Life*

Praise for
MIND BODY F.I.T. METHOD

"Mind Body FIT is an awesome support to release what's holding me back from my healthiest self. De'Anna is a wonderful friend and mentor. Priceless, beautiful, self loving nurturing."

Carole Christmas Hoffer, MA FACMPE
University Medical Group, Greenville Health System

"Where to start? Well, it started in 2011, joining Mind Body FIT to achieve a healthy mindset. Then followed by coaching for my first half marathon in 2013, straight into private coaching. The gifts and tools DeAnna have given me through the years have changed my life. I make sure to tell her often and from my heart, "I don't know where I'd be in my life right now if it wasn't for you!" My love and gratitude for our years of work together are beyond measure, "priceless!"

Jennifer Quinlan,
NYC Model, Actor, Domestic Violence Advocacy

"Mind Body FIT is an amazing group of women who get it! They understand the ins and outs of weight loss and weight gain and the things in life that can affect those drastic changes. Founder De'Anna Nunez is a wealth of information and provides valuable tools that dramatically change the way you see yourself and love who you are today! She guides her clients to a healthy mental state clearing the way for productive weight loss and longevity in healthy lifestyle living. I love MBFC for all it has given me and the tools I never had before, I'm proud to be a lifelong MBFC lady!"

Genelle Rich
Top Performing Realtor and Business Leader,
Easterby & Associates Keller Williams

"The committed people in the Mind Body FIT Community and the authenticity of the comments inside the group have touched my heart! I always come away feeling loved, listened to and like I belong. De'Anna has created and holds together this beautiful space with her unique skills that literally get our minds in a space that is sustainable for life. We are all challenged at our own pace, but watching everyone's growth adds to my own. The honesty and compassion inside the community blows me away! Getting rid of the diet culture is a continuing theme and it is a perfect fit for me. De'Anna's effervescence is contagious! Come join us!"

RaNae Bennett
Retired School Teacher, Writer, Creator
of Analogies of Nature

"In 2010 when I met this amazing woman, DeAnna Nunez, little did I know she would become the catalyst for complete change in my life. At the time I was feeling naked, vulnerable and out of control. She gave me the courage I needed to push myself to try again to lose the weight I had carried my whole adult life and the "I CAN" mindset to lose over 100 lbs and maintain it for over 7 years!"

Jaylene Welch
Top Sales and Customer Care at Precision Plastic Surgery

"Most people who want to lose weight know what they need to do, but they don't know why they can't do it. In this book, De'Anna Nunez explains exactly what the obstacles are. She provides achievable steps to changing your life patterns, so that you feel better every single day, creating health and happiness that lasts!"

Alegra Loewenstein,
Author of Emotional Eating Detox

"De'Anna Nunez is the light! She is the real deal. She lives what she preaches. Mind, Body Fitness! De'Anna literally helped me gain perspectives on all these areas of my life. I was stuck on why I couldn't get healthy. She gave me the necessary tools I needed for my breakthroughs! So far I am 17.7 lbs healthier and looking forward to more. Love this gal for saving my life. She carries such wisdom, caring, and a loving spirit. I thank God for her as she has helped me with my journey to not only get to my healthy self, but also for my business. She gives tools and resources that really work. XoXo."

Martha Munoz
CEO of MedCare, Founder of Women's Legacy
of Hope, Author of Hiding From Myself

"I've had the honor of having De'Anna help me through private sessions of dealing with internal issues that weighed on me for years. I successfully conquered my issues! Today I can say I'm darn proud of what I've accomplished in my life and also the courage to dig deep and change my internal voice. Thanks girlie!"

Donna Davis
Successfully Retired, Beachbum

"So much time is wasted in today's diet culture – counting calories, judging ourselves harshly, trying to trick ourselves into complying with anything that improves how we look. Here, De'Anna teaches a compassionate and mindful way to love ourselves into releasing weight. Anyone stuck in any type of cycle, whether it be poor eating, addictions or negative self-talk would benefit from this fresh approach to living our most vital life!"

RaNae Bennett
Retired School Teacher, Writer, Creator
of Analogies of Nature

"De'Anna's a spot on role model!"

Lauren Albrecht
Adventure Guide Concierge, Mammoth Mountain

"It is hard to live the life of your dreams when you don't feel good in your body. That's why De'Anna Nunez is the perfect person to deliver MIND BODY FIT LIFE to the world ... to you. For as long as I have known her, De'Anna has LIVED her methodology in the most beautiful and profound way—in her personal AND professional life. And she demonstrates that taking care of your health overflows into EVERY area of your life. Plus, she has studied the subconscious mind for 20 years and KNOWS how to help YOU make the mental shift you need to discover—and keep— the beautiful and fit body that is waiting to be unveiled."

Ursula Mentjes,
Award Winning Author and Entrepreneur

DE'ANNA NUNEZ

MIND BODY F.I.T. *Life*

Activate your Subconscious Power

**for weight release, self belief,
emotional eating and fully
embodying a healthy mindset**

savvygirlpress
• • •

ISBN 978-0-9838684-1-5 paperback
ISBN 978-0-9838684-2-2 ebook

Library of Congress Cataloging-in-Publishing Data is available upon request. Printed in the United States of America

First Printing, 2020

Edited by Bonnie Gruttadauria with Get Branded Press
Cover & Interior Design by Kateryna Korniienko-Heidtman

Dedication

This book is dedicated to my Mom, Nancy Jo Dermid. You are home.

And, to my loving family. Troy, Zach, Janelle, Vasco, Savvy, Diane, Jeanette, Carlene, Jessica, Hannah, Rick, Cecil, Doug, Dad, Terri, Debbie.

Special Acknowledgments

To my family. You are my everything.

And, to the awe-inspiring women who have taught me resilience, courage and self value. You are so bad-ass. Your willingness to explore necessary healing, be vulnerable and carry-on stronger is a gift I value greatly. May we all continue to rise.

Table of Contents

Foreword
by Nichole MacDonald

When I was a kid, I thought I'd have it all figured out when I grew up. I'd have a boyfriend and bouncy hair and high heels and a cool job. I'd eat whatever I wanted because nobody could tell me no.

I'd figure out how to do a smooth ponytail, like the mystical girl who sat in front of me in class. How did she do that, anyway? She'll grow up and make everything look easy. She will have a boyfriend with an accent and he'll pick her up and swing her around and they'll giggle loudly and smooch.

We all know that girl. She grew up, too. She's the one who still won't eat a piece of your kid's birthday cake because she's too full from her celery juice. She doesn't have self sabotaging behaviors or cravings or a muffin top. Why is her life so easy?

Of course, as grown ups we realize that we actually have no idea what is going on with anyone, sometimes not even ourselves. Smooth ponytail girl's mom might have held impossible standards and maybe she grew up to perpetuate the same unhealthy expectations. Maybe she's just really good at ponytails.

But this book is not about ponytails. It's about all the silly and amazing and destructive and powerful ways you control your own life and outcomes. It's about getting over yourself and the way you thought things were going to go. It's about ditching your limiting beliefs to create the life you want for yourself. It's about using the power of your mind for good, not evil. And it's written by the queen of bumpy ponytails, my dear friend, De'Anna Nunez.

De'Anna spent much of her life struggling like the rest of us. She gets it. All of it. She approaches transformation with humor, lightness, and a clarity that has you wonder how you didn't see these things before. And a reminder that, it's okay that you didn't! Because neither did I! And neither did she... until she did.

I first reached out to De'Anna because I didn't have it all figured out. I built a multi-million dollar business, but I couldn't keep my house organized or my mouth from consuming copious amounts of sugar. The thing I love most about De'Anna is you can take literally any problem to her—anything—and she'll use her magic wand to turn it into something empowering. Then she hands you the magic wand.

As you read this book, I want you to imagine yourself hanging out with De'Anna. She is the girlfriend relentlessly by your side, who has mastered the mysterious ways of the smooth ponytail girls, and is giving us all the juicy details. She cares about you so much, it's almost annoying.

She is relentless in her stand for you. She will hold you accountable to what you say you want in your life. She will stand up for you when you won't stand up for yourself.

She rocks her bumpy ponytail and drinks her celery juice and also eats your kid's birthday cake. She shares a bottle of wine with you and then makes you run up a mountain with her. She is the one who makes it easy because it was never hard to begin with. We just made it hard with all the disempowering stories we were telling ourselves. She's telling you a new one.

Take it in. Then take it on.

Get your magic wand.

We'll see you at the top of the mountain.

Introduction

I See YOU. You are part of a growing tribe of women who want to lead your life with more confidence. Feeling good in your body is an important aspect of that journey and you've got a nagging voice in the back of your head that is urging you to pay more attention. You have the desire to live a healthy lifestyle, yet on the inside you may feel like you're falling behind. Truth is, sometimes you're chilling out after long days by rewarding yourself with food, a media binge, or both, even though you know a walk to de-stress would be a better choice.

Admittedly, living your full dream doesn't seem quite possible without also being your healthiest and most vibrant. I mean ... that's part of the dream too, right? Do you think you must let go of certain foods, or exercise like crazy, to reach and maintain your ideal weight? It's not true. We've just been messed up in the mind by unrealistic expectations and the diet mindset our culture has fed us. It's time to let all that go, because it's not just about the external stuff—food, exercise, cleanses and bootcamps. It's not even about how much you weigh. It's about YOU.

The journey to your promised land, the place where you can maintain a healthy body and perform to the level of life's demands without sacrificing your health, is where we are headed together in this book. You will learn how to experience your full vibrant health and it starts by way of internal design.

F.I.T. is an acronym for Focus, Inward, Target. It's a method. Think of the F.I.T. Method as advanced creative problem-solving, rewiring your mind, clearing out unwanted subconscious baggage, and reinforcing your innate strengths and values so deeply, it's as if it sinks into your bones.

My goal is to be the wisdom-whisperer in your head that feeds you positive solutions. I will show you how to utilize your subconscious mind to release extra pounds without dieting and how to make tiny, easy changes to your thinking habits that will make all the difference. You will be learning and integrating a version of self-hypnosis that I have spent years refining. Essentially, instead of looking outside for the answers, you'll learn a method for looking within and deeply trusting yourself.

Every day you are hypnotizing yourself with your own recycled thinking. Your very thoughts perpetuate and fixate on circumstances, fears and the residue of the past. Even when you create exciting plans for your healthier future, the goals you didn't reach and the imprints of past emotional situations influence your thinking and feed in you thoughts of self doubt.

I'm going to teach you the mindset skills to change everything. Just imagine how glorious it will be when you're walking in your freedom and know exactly how to navigate more triumphantly in your future.

This amazing work I feel so blessed to share with you will teach you how to let go. Your subconscious is holding on to food habits and body beliefs that do not support you.

My professional experience knows, the food is not the real problem. It's not even about the weight either. It's the undercurrent happening below the surface, in your subconscious, that weighs heavy.

Sometimes you may place blame on the external stuff—your job, a relationship, an unsettling circumstance or your schedule. All of those things make it hard for you to concentrate on getting healthy. But the real issue is the program playing in the background of your mind. It needs to be changed.

You know you could be much more in control, but you're not always exercising that mindset muscle, and often, your own thinking is getting in the way and sabotaging you. Habitual overthinking patterns are stressful—and it probably drives you crazy when you do that. Overthinking what it will take to get healthy only stalls your progress more.

The effects of internal stressors go deeper than you may realize and learning to consciously manage your mind is an essential practice. In this book, I intend to make you conscious of what is currently unconscious for you; reveal the mental blocks and bathe you in your true essence. One client recently said, "De'Anna, you helped me connect the dots as to why I was doing what I was doing. It felt like a revelation!"

I know the mind-body journey from a multidimensional perspective and because of that, I know you'll find this book to be superbly helpful. I've personally experienced how liberating it is to overcome the internal struggle.

I've now been able to sustain a healthy body weight for a number of years as a result of my own breakthrough. I discovered the extra benefits that go beyond aesthetics are a true sense of internal belief, peace within, confidence and the mindset that you can do anything.

What makes all the difference? It's your thinking habits and the connection they have to your unconscious mind. You may think sugar cravings are the real issue. Or do you think salty, crunchy food was your biggest problem? I can tell you, those things are not the real problem. They are just the symptom of the problem. We'll get underneath it in this book and free you forever. New beneficial thinking habits will allow you to shed unnecessary pounds without having to try so hard.

They say you don't become an expert until you've reached 10,000 hours. I have those 10,000 hours invested in practicing, educating and facilitating the F.I.T. Method and you're about to benefit. Know that my advice is sound and based in scientific research. I will share expertise from my professional experience as a Hypnotist, having hypnotized over 10,000 people and having taught hypnosis to over 500,000 audience members.

Through the exercises in this book, my goal is to help you create a breakthrough (or multiple breakthroughs). I'll teach you how beliefs and thinking habits are birthed and how to reframe them to shift your subconscious mind and realign with new habits. I would love to see you go from bouts of unbeneficial stress, worry, overwhelm, inadequacy, insecurity or fear—to beneficial, supportive thinking habits that gracefully hold self-love and trust in yourself at the core. I'll help you to stop talking yourself out of exercise or turning to food for the wrong reasons and how to step into your greatness like it's a magical snap of your fingers.

The psychological aspects of designing a healthy lifestyle are the key components to your success. Truly, within you are all the pieces to the puzzle, the pieces may just be out of position. Most people do not realize they already hold the key, but in this book, I'll draw it out of you. And you'll see how all the pieces fit perfectly, like the mosaic you are.

We'll change things up. When embarking on a lifestyle change, typically, people turn to an eating plan as if it holds all the power, or they make a commitment to exercise and jump in with both feet. Yes, those are things you do to live a healthy lifestyle, but to truly sustain your habits with greater ease longterm, you must form an internal foundation of subconscious belief and self-identity. You must adopt a new agreement with your mind and body to believe this is who you are.

In this book, you'll dare to get outside your current vision of yourself and dream a new dream. Imagine being F.I.T. and how that will empower you to show up in your career with more confidence and boldness. Imagine being F.I.T. and your relationships improve because your insecurities are in check and you know exactly who you are. Because you've taken charge of yourself, you're a better leader, and perhaps you'll even make more money with less stress as a result.

My client Jaylene Welch shed over 100 pounds in 13 months without a bar, shake or specific meal plan. Included with that release, was letting go of an unhappy marriage. As she explored her deepest truths and accepted herself, her self-confidence skyrocketed. This was not a direct result from the weight loss, but from who she became in the interim. She also quit her job and found a new one that paid her twice the amount. You see, the benefits that accompany self-exploration are hugely prosperous.

Throughout this book, I urge you to explore inward and make new decisions to align yourself with your most fulfilling vision for your life. I lay out the framework, step-by-step, and you make the all-important mindset shift happen.

By now you might have discovered what this book is NOT about. It's not a book about a butt lift exercise that will give you a model-like backside (as great as that may be). It's not about specific foods that will help you feel less bloated. It's about YOU. Throughout these pages you'll discover real life stories that attach to mindset models with proven success. You'll also connect with the most vulnerable parts of yourself. It will peel you like an onion and absolutely propel you to a new way of living F.I.T. and healthy.

You deserve nothing short of a spectacular life. No more putting on a happy face, while behind the scenes feeling incomplete. No more forcing yourself to compartmentalize or ignore painful or stressful aspects of your life. With courage, you'll uncover what you've been avoiding and now work towards total fulfillment.

You'll be shocked at just how much those things have been unconsciously affecting you.

This book was written to heal, share, and cause you to create new thinking habits between your mind and body. Neuroscientist Dr. Leaf says, "Your body is not in control of your mind—your mind is in control of your body, and your mind is stronger than your body." I'll help you release the obsessiveness with food, weight and dieting, yet still reach your healthiest, sustainable weight. I'm here to provide the framework for that breakthrough. It begins with your mind. Together, we will create a treaty between your thoughts and your body's receptors.

So often, when I'm asking a new client about her health goals, she'll recall stories of how she *used to be* and express a desire to be like that again. Hold up! You are in a new season of life. You can't go back, there's only forward. And hey, you're wiser now than you were 20 ago or even 10 years ago. You're better than before regardless of where you are in your weight. It's vital that we align your mind and body with the most powerful moment in time. That's NOW.

Plato said, "An unexamined life is not worth living." You and I will do some necessary cultivating; we'll pull the weeds and plant new seeds so you can move forward most powerfully. Your journey with this book will guide you to examine the inside, because it's the command center of all that is possible for you. Our goal will be to bring the best lessons from your past, and apply them as values in the here and now. My values-based exercise is one of my clients' favorite processes. They love how it shifts their thinking! I share with you in this book the very process I use with my one-on-one clients who invest in programs with me.

To receive the most from this book, I encourage you to proceed as if you are an explorer! The **F.I.T.** journey courageously explores Focusing Inward and Targeting key aspects of your inner self. Throughout the chapters are the very components that will free you from the vicious cycle of dieting or inconsistency with your health.

You will experience ...

- An exploration of your deepest fear
  with a brave and courageous heart.

- Unmet needs—so you can stop merely
  coping, and actually be fulfilled.

- Your subconscious associations with food, your
  body and other things you've deemed important.

- Designing a grander vision of who you are
  or want to be in regards to your health.

- Self-trust as a bridge to becoming
  your best vision of healthy.

- A deep connection to why it matters
  that you actually do it.

- Adopting a never-give-up attitude.

- And more ...

I will uncover how deep beliefs and behaviors are formed, and you'll discover how significantly they may have subconsciously affected you. You may not be presently conscious of the root cause. But by sharing professional insights and coaching frameworks with you, I know that you will make a bright new connection and step into your future-self more brilliantly.

For any of us who have slacked on taking care of ourselves, have used food and/or wine as a friend, partner, ally or enemy, you know that it doesn't take much turmoil or a trigger to turn to the fridge or cupboards for comfort. Yet, through the psychological and emotional development prompts in this book, you will make the connection and overcome behaviors that are not really serving you.

It is from an empathetic and compassionate state of mind that you can build a strong, healthy body and a healthy life you can love living. That strength and confidence will allow you to lead in the workplace, create better relationships with food, money and people, and truly feel fulfilled. Wholehearted living is what I want for you.

First you must ask yourself, *Am I willing?* Willingness is the entry point of all self-growth. Are you willing to take a compassionate look at yourself and make the vital changes that you know will make all the difference? I'll ask you to up your willingness game.

Secondly, why does it matter that you take action? Together, I'll help you unpack your deeper purpose for getting F.I.T. Your big WHY must go beyond fitting into your skinny jeans, otherwise you'd just be on another diet, and you won't stay motivated long enough to have the necessary breakthroughs required for sustainability.

I have divided the book in sections to align with a framework of three guiding principles. DESIRE. COURAGE. ACTION. These three principles have been the foundation for women in my Mind Body F.I.T. Community and have led them to let go of limiting beliefs, unhealthy paradigms and take charge of their health in a myriad of powerful new ways.

In the framework I've provided, you'll discover the bravery to really go for it. As a professional Hypnotherapist, I will guide you to explore your mind from a safe and compassionate perspective, and encourage you to have the courage to look within. I believe by reconnecting to yourself, you'll discover your dreams and inspiration again to live healthy. And this time it will be even more amazing because ... this process is 100% Anti-Diet.

In section one, DESIRE, I urge you to want what you want. To fully give yourself permission to matter in all facets of who you are. We often define ourselves by our achievements or our sacrifices as if they are a measure of why we are worth what we're worth. I will ask you to go beyond circumstance and take ownership of why you really matter. Beyond your accolades. I want you to connect with the essence and spirit that you bring to the world. That thing that makes you, YOU, is your worth. Your body is the container of that precious gift. I'll ask you to become more willing to nurture and value that vessel.

In section two, COURAGE, we'll explore what it really means to be courageous. Jumping out of a plane may be the first vision in your mind when you associate with courageousness, but the type of courage I'm asking of you is within yourself. To explore those parts of you that you've ignored or suppressed. The stuff you've pushed way deep down are often your gems, but they need to be unmined and refined to see their brilliance. If you've got stuff that you thought you dealt with, yet you're still struggling with weight or lack of motivation, my professional expertise says, it is not resolved on a subconscious level. I guarantee you, your weight is not the problem, it is the by-product of the problem, and only your subconscious has the solution. It's time you get courageous, do some mining, and I guarantee you'll discover a vein of precious gemstones.

In section three, I'll invite you to put your wisdom to use and train your mind to ACT on your new thinking. I plan to get you fired up! Knowledge is the key, but action unlocks the lock. You absolutely must practice what you internally learn. I will show you how to systemize your habits, create motivation on demand, blow through fears with greater ease and talk to yourself with a more beneficial language. I'll even show you how to design affirmations that actually work! All of these actions will keep you out of the dark rabbit hole and move forward with consistency. Perhaps in the past you've put forth effort toward being healthy, but you couldn't sustain it. Now you'll be able to show up your best every day.

Throughout the back and at the end of each chapter you'll be invited to participate in a F.I.T. Exercise. As a Hypnotist, my expertise is focused on exploring the down, and I couldn't understand what she was physically dying from. I mean, I knew she was unhealthy, but she didn't have a disease or an exact issue of concern that could kill you. When I asked the doctor, he said, "Well, essentially poor self-care." In the end she died of the very issue my crusade was meant to prevent; a woman not valuing herself enough to take care of her mental, emotional and physical health.

You're here and reading this book. You are ready to make changes. The effort you make heals Mom's journey in so many ways *(thank you)* and makes it worth the many long hours I've spent pouring into these chapters. I absolutely love this mind-body journey and I love you for being the type of person who sees the value in investing your time and energy into making your life a magnificent adventure.

I'm here to lead you and support you to succeed. Sometimes I'll call you out and tell you the God's-honest truth. Other times, I'll hug you with words and remind you of how awesome you are. Your struggle is the struggle of many. You are not alone. In this environment you are surrounded by women who have shifted their mind-body struggle into one of strength. It's a methodology you can depend on moving forward and a contagious, optimistic attitude that is sure to open your mind and heart. Let's agree that from here forward you will make optimism your oxygen.

Who You Are Becoming

The new F.I.T. you is brave and courageous with your emotions and yourself. You are willing to explore your deepest fears. You are willing to show up for yourself with acceptance, love and compassion. You see the benefit of your true needs being met and know that feeling good goes beyond wine, frozen yogurt, pizza or getting your nails done.

You are a woman with a vision and a determination to fulfill and live that vision. It matters that you take this journey to ultimate well-being. You value meaning in your life and have come to learn that all the struggles have artistically shaped the mosaic of who you are today. Fearlessness has taken on a new essence. You know you need to trust yourself more deeply in each step. You approach life like a warrior, willing to battle for what and who you believe in. You do not fight small fights of frivolous nonsense or ignorance. You lead with integrity.

You are learning that your body matters. It is the reflection of your heart and habits and is the very vehicle that allows you to show up to your life with joy. You take risks within yourself and for the greater good of your vision. You have adopted a never-give-up attitude in other areas of your life and are learning to trust yourself in an abundance of ways. You are a badass. You are a rebel. The new you says, "I am here to make my mark and to live a full life." I know that woman. She is you. She is me.

In the opening chapter, I'll expose the mysterious powers of the subconscious mind so that they are not so mysterious. I'll teach you how to use the F.I.T. Method to reshape your mind, clear out the clutter and view your body with gratitude and fierce strength. Let's get started.

Getting Started

My vision for you is to use this book as a hybrid tool. I see you experiencing *omg moments* as you read, breakthroughs as you interact and opportunities of self-growth as you partner with me through the meaningful concepts, stories and exercises.

- Don't just read it as a book, internalize the parts that resonate and take action

- Interact with it as a journal by writing down your thoughts as you go

- Invest in yourself by experiencing the visualization and F.I.T. exercises

5 Things You Must Know Before You Make Any Weight Loss Goals

There are traps that make weight release harder than it needs to be and you've probably fallen into them from time to time. Attune your mind to new thinking and you'll be able to live life as the badass you are with eyes wide open. Do not let the old way of diet-thinking fog your clarity.

5 Weight Release Traps

#1 We focus on the meal plan we're following, not the good habits we're building.

Have you ever heard you and your friends say something like this?

Hey Lisa, you look great, what are you doing?

Oh I'm on _____, it's great you should try it. It works.

We give our power away. Truth is, you are what worked, not just the diet. Because you put time, effort and focus into what you're eating, you got results. That's not the diet's victory, that's yours! Yet, we tend to give all the credit to the diet and not ourselves.

As soon as we stop focusing on the regimen, we stop working. We don't blame the diet, we blame ourselves and then we start the diet over when we are motivated again. But that is often after weeks or months of what we consider blowing it or getting off-track. That's a hard process to put yourself through repeatedly.

#2 We focus on what we can't have.

Deprivation leads the way in most diets. When our excitement to lose weight gets us motivated and focused, the first thing we do is prepare our minds and kitchens for a life without our favorite foods. If we do allow them, it is on a minimal basis.

The deprivation mindset messes with our focus and we find ourselves often fixated on what we cannot have, especially in moments of emotional charge (such as celebrations, work and family stress or relationship issues). In that moment, try to NOT think about eating your favorite foods and you'll just focus on them more. Go ahead, DON'T think about your food now (chips, ice cream, wine). Don't think about it. Just don't. See what I mean? Your mind does not hear "NOT." It's even harder in those shaky emotional moments.

#3 We focus on a period of time or an end date.

We often start a diet because of a special day that is weeks or months down the road. A date, a wedding, a job interview, a high school reunion, your birthday ... all reasons why we start dieting. Dieting causes a start and stop mindset that entraps us. We stay focused just for a period of time. We win the day but not the lifetime. We soon find ourselves back on a diet when we notice we've been slacking or our pants don't fit again.

#4 We underestimate the power of habit.

Weight loss is hard because our subconscious mind is on default mode and simply repeating patterns that have been practiced and engrained for years. When we make a decision to lose weight, we are often underestimating the power of those old patterns, and we don't stick with our eating habits long enough to override them. We also get stuck in habit loops. That includes the habit loop of dieting. When we start, our subconscious mind already knows it will soon end, because that's the pattern. We'll keep looping and starting again, like a hamster on a wheel or the definition of insanity – doing the same thing over and over expecting a different result.

#5 We don't look beyond food and exercise.

We make losing and maintaining hard when we are unwilling to look at the emotional subsets that have kept us turning to food for the wrong reasons. Our subconscious mind has created emotional associations with food and until you realize it's not about the actual food, but what the food means to you, you will find it very difficult to keep off any weight you've lost.

Understanding the reason WHY weight has been an issue is what makes losing it easy this time! Once you know your WHY, stop asking it and just get to taking action. We can loop ourselves into a trap asking why for too long when we very well know the answer.

PART 1

DESIRE FOR BETTER

Chapter 1

The F.I.T. Method as Your Superpower

Whatever we plant in our subconscious
mind and nourish with repetition and
emotion will one day become a reality.
~ Earl Nightengale

Imagine tapping into a state of mind that has zero percent self doubt. As if you are unstoppable! How much further along would you be toward your dreams, goals and aspirations by accessing that power?

That is the F.I.T. Method. It is a mindset you can learn to impregnate your goals and uplevel your life. The very goals you've got floating in the back of your head or maybe even written down in your favorite journal or smartphone; you could utilize this superpower state of mind to infuse a deep belief that you will 100% achieve them. This phenomenal mindset also has the ability to break through the stuff that causes resistance along the way, making it that much faster to create momentum.

Think of the F.I.T. Method as neuroscience in action. It is an advanced creative problem-solving, clearing out unwanted subconscious baggage and reinforcing your innate strengths and values. Essentially, instead of looking outside for the answers, you'll learn a method for looking within and deeply trusting yourself. The idealogy is based in emotional proficiency, kinesthetics, behavioral science, psychology and an advanced version of self-hypnosis and HNLP (Humanisitic Neuro Linguistic Pscyhology). I've combined these incredible methods in an effort to provoke subconscious change for you. The F.I.T. Method will enable you to tap your internal resources and redesign them for your success.

You don't need another guru's blueprint for success when you can design your own. Within these pages, my goal is to expose you to a new way of interacting with your mind and emotions and teach you communication skills between your conscious and subconscious mind so you can be happy and sustainable in your weight for many years to come.

WHY HIGH PERFORMANCE HYPNOSIS

As a trained professional Hypnotist and Instructor of Hypnosis, I use the technique of putting a client into a heightened state of concentration and focus on their most positive outcome. Together, we tap into your own brain wave superpowers.

The definition of hypnosis is a natural state of consciousness experienced as heightened awareness or deep relaxation. It is is being utilized in the medical field as a first-line intervention for stress-related illnesses, pain management, weight loss, smoking cessation, dementia, PTSD, mental health and more. There are hospitals and medical clinics throughout the world with trained professional hypnotists, like myself, on staff to work with patients.

Beyond medical interventions, it is used as a peak performance tool for athletes, executive training and team building. I've been blessed to work with Olympians referred through their sports medicine physician to improve focus, release from distraction and create positive mental imagery. I even helped a pro soccer player release his fear of flying as he traveled from game to game.

You experience hypnosis every day on your own but don't necessarily realize that's what you're experiencing. For instance, I mentioned driving in the car, arriving at your destination and not remembering the drive. That is a light state of hypnosis. You've done that. Think about it, you've driven across town, passed your exit by accident and don't even remember the last 20 minutes. Your conscious mind wandered around your thoughts, while your subconscious drove the car. You learned to drive years ago and therefore now no longer need your cognitive state to know how to drive. All the information is stored subconsciously.

In my work, I utilize the natural abilities of the mind for you to experience mental imagery and attach verbal cues to deepen the connection you have with your own psychological processes. Neuroscience shows us that we can actually grow new neuropathways using these methods. Your brain can change! Imagine how useful that is to the way you view, interact, talk to and behave in your body.

I became enamored with the science of mind in my 20s and I used hypnosis as a tool to help myself overcome psychological obstacles that I felt held me back. Essentially, that means I had stuff in the back of my head that I wanted to get rid of so I could be more successful in life! Throughout this book you'll learn more of my story, but for now, I really want to dive into the process of the F.I.T. Method so that you can be educated on what it is, how it works, and start implementing it into your weight shed journey.

Science and modern technology can now prove hypnosis. If we hooked you up to an EEG, a medical technology used to measure brain activity, during a F.I.T. Hypnosis experience, we could see your brain waves engaging with the process. The imagery you would see is your brain slowing down into higher states of focus. It's intriguing to watch and also takes some of the mystery out of it.

Hypnosis is proven to occur within the brain waves of alpha and theta, right before you drift off to sleep. Now, as you read the words on this page, you are most likely in a beta state, which means you are alert and focusing on an external stimulus. In a beta state, you are utilizing the front lobe of your brain and processing analytically. We generally refer to this as the conscious mind.

As you engage in the F.I.T. Method's self-hypnosis prompts, the goal is to drop into alpha and theta states. This state of mind shows specific changes in brain activity that can be positive interventions for new thought. These states of consciousness are something your mind does regularly without you realizing it like daydreaming in class as a young student, driving across town or having an answer or solution pop into your mind while showering.

You can utilize these brain waves to influence the subconscoius. You can speak, feel, communicate and re-learn patterns in your mind so that you can make healthy beliefs and habits your new normal.

Here's how your brain waves work:

BETA: External stimulus, focused attention (like you reading this book right now)

ALPHA: Dreamy, super-learning, imagination, effortless relaxation (eyes open hypnosis – walking, hiking, driving, painting, showering etc.)

THETA: Intuition, meditation, insight, deep emotional connection, dreaming (typically eyes closed hypnosis – inner focus, intuitive hits, deeper concentration)

DELTA: Deep REM sleep

The alpha and theta waves are what we designate as states of hypnosis, whereas you are either deeply relaxed, or intensely focused on new learning and open to new ideas and suggestions. It is within this state of mind you can present the brain with new options and interrupt lifelong patterns that have been previously established. We also know the subconscious mind is not just in the brain. It encompasses the entire nervous system and is unconsciously communicating between mind and body. There is an interconnectedness that has been proven and thoroughly researched. You can take advantage of the genius that is already within you, and leverage its capabilities to help you be your healthiest.

I encourage you to release any earlier judgements or misconceptions you may have had about Hypnosis. Those that say Hypnosis is evil or controlling are simply, terribly misinformed and perhaps fearful of what they don't comprehend. Understandably, it has been overdramatized in movies and often misinterpreted. It is a fallacy that you go under another's control. Instead, think of it as going into your own brain waves and experiencing what they were created to do. It has always been my intention from the beginning of my career to showcase Hypnosis in positive ways, and not just tell you, but show you the magnificent effects of learning Hypnotic processes. The results speak for themselves by way of our Mind Body F.I.T. community members sharing weight shed stories, burdens they've let go of and truths they now live by.

In the F.I.T. Method, you are increasing your ability to manage your mind more effectively and positively. Have you experienced being stuck in overthinking patterns (monkey mind) and it steals your ability to stay focused on a goal? Perhaps you overthink exercise. It's on your mind with good intentions, you keep thinking about it, but you don't actually do it. The F.I.T. Method will be phenomenal for you.

Your mind solely belongs to you. It's like the captain of your ship. You may have had times in your life where your mind was influenced by tough circumstances or people. Like a ship navigating a storm, you cannot control the weather, but you can control how you respond to the weather. Our work begins by you grasping this next important concept. All thought patterns that become the way you think about yourself are created by your own willingness to accept them. I invite you to explore your mind to discover what's been blocking your success. Aristotle said, "Knowing yourself is the beginning of all wisdom." It's from that point of view that I ask you to delve into this process wholeheartedly. Your mind is more powerful than you've been giving it credit. Once you learn to focus its abilities toward your good, there is nothing you cannot accomplish.

A FEW WAYS I'VE SUCCESSFULLY USED SELF-HYPNOSIS

I have personally used the F.I.T. Method's self-hypnosis techniques to birth two of my babies with no pain. During the entire birthing process, I maintained an alpha-theta state by focusing inward and targeting a specific state of relaxed mind. The goal was to deeply trust my body and allow it to do what it instinctively knows. No clenching or tightening from fear. Instead, loose, limp and relaxed.

The verbal cue 'surrender' was a word I used every time I inhaled and exhaled deeply. Using mental imagery, I imagined opening up and giving way to the baby making its journey into life. I also used the phenomenon of deep, hypnotic suggestion to block pain. I experienced discomfort cues as pressure and contractions as waves. It felt like a lot of pressure, but no pain. Beautifully, I was able to experience the entire birthing process without even a Tylenol. It was amazing.

I am so thankful for The Hypnobabies Program, created by renowned Registered Nurse and Hypnotist Karrie Tuschoff. Becoming a Certified Hypnobabies Instructor helped me to birth my own baby peacefully, and without unnecessary medical interventions that used to be standard practice in many hospitals. Luckily, hospital administrators are shifting their mindset and now entire birthing centers are staffed with nurses that are trained in hypnosis.

Another time I used hypnosis on the fly while in a disheartening and unexpected situation. I accidentally broke a glass vase and the sharp edges slit through my thumb severing my tendon inside. The wound was deep, and I knew it would require stitches. I used the F.I.T. Method to go to a calm, peaceful place so I could maintain composure in front of my toddlers. I didn't want to freak them out! I gave myself the hypnotic suggestion to engage in visual imagery. I imagined a dam at my wrist, pooling the blood there to prevent further bleeding. It worked so beautifully that I was able to successfully walk into the emergency room with no bleeding whatsoever. When the nurse asked me my pain level, I said, "None, I'm practicing self-hypnosis." Ha! She looked at me with her mouth dropped open. It was so cool.

I invite you to look deeper into the power of this method. You'll discover over 290,000 academic papers on Google Scholar and thousands of cases where hypnosis was used positively to overcome an array of issues. It's being used at the Mayo Clinic, UCLA Children's Hospital and many top universities such as Harvard and Stanford. It is safe and viable. As shared here, hypnosis is a powerful tool that you have access to at any given moment, and can be utilized in a number of ways. In the chapters to come, I'll be teaching you how to apply this method as an extraordinary communication tool between your mind and body. We'll be combining relaxation and visualization techniques with coaching prompts to create a fresh new internal dialogue of belief and confidence in yourself.

Consider ... you have been in your own hypnosis for

years. The thoughts you think and the habits you keep were designed and shaped by you. Your own perpetual, internal recycling of thoughts have kept you entrapped in a line of thinking held by your own subconscious paradigms. It's become so ingrained, it's unconscious. It feels tough to change because it's below the surface and often elusive. You may have been unclear on what specifically needs to be rewired. Until now.

THE INNER WORKINGS OF THE F.I.T. METHOD

As there are a large variety of ways to experience self-hypnosis, I will teach you my protocols. There is eyes open Hypnosis and can be utilized while in motion as a focused concentration tool. It is this method that is popular amongst peak performance athletes. I've used it myself in many marathons. I've fended off cramps, stayed connected to my vision or recited a mantra from mind to body as a committed effort to encompass supermind abilities into those tough moments. It works! I'll be offering up the eyes open technique throughout the book.

Right now I'd like to start with incorporating the practice of deep reflection and rewire method. It is not necessary to be lying down but can be helpful in order to achieve a relaxed state of mind. Many of my clients that I hypnotize over the phone in my Breakthrough Sessions enjoy being in their bed, on the couch or a comfy chair. This is a foundational process that you'll interact with throughout the book to accelerate your growth. Keep in mind that it can be practiced anywhere, anytime. I urge you to not use it while driving.

Prepare your space for quiet. Interruptions can distract you, therefore, to receive a higher level of benefit, turn off your phone and close the door. You will not fall asleep, even though it can emulate the feeling of drifting off. You'll soon experience a meditative state of stillness and calm. The biggest difference between hypnosis and meditation is that hypnosis is for the purpose of achieving a goal whereas meditation's purpose is to simply be.

Now before I lead you through this, I have to share that it is entirely possible to experience hypnosis with people all around you. For instance, my presentations are in front of 50-10,000 audience members. Even with people watching, my participants can focus and enter into hypnosis. At one part of my career, I performed 303 shows for a theme park as a headlining act. My stage was amphitheater style, open to the sky, with a fast and loud roller coaster furiously swooshing by. I always took volunteers from the audience, and even with that roaring roller coaster passing by every three minutes filled with screaming riders, people on my stage still went into hypnosis fabulously. So you see, your mind is powerful when you focus it.

Practice getting good at the F.I.T. Method while interacting with all the questions and exercises in this book. Use the process to:

- Observe yourself from an objective perspective

- Disrupt overthinking or old patterns

- Internalize your goals (let'em
  soak into your muscle)

- Let go of emotional pain or struggle

- Interact with your creative, colorful mind

- Deeply connect with a new gratitude
  for your body and mind

- Instill healthy thinking habit patterns

- Trust yourself more deeply, and connect
  to that essence and feeling more often

Let's create a practice session now. To begin, start with your heart. For 25 years much study has been conducted at the HeartMath Institute in Colorado showing significant evidence on the improvement of emotional well-being through the heart-brain connection. With over 300 peer reviewed scientific studies, evidence shows that within two minutes, by engaging your thought connection with your heart, you can create coherence and feelings of well-being.

*Read through the entire process
first, then come back to Step 1
to implement and practice.*

The F.I.T. Method's Advanced
Self-Hypnosis Process

— Step 1 —

For those of you who experience monkey mind or the inability to release from mental distraction, this part of the F.I.T. Method is imperative for you to learn. You'll love how it quickly and easily helps you to zero in and become focused.

Begin by placing your dominant hand on your heart. Choose a focal point. Fixate your eyes on a particular spot. It can be on the ceiling or across the room. Don't take your eyes from that spot, even if you feel the urge to look around. Fixate. This technique helps you to fend off distractions and tells your mind it's time to focus.

— Step 2 —

Begin practicing deep breathing. Take in a full deep breath, hold it at the top for 4-5 seconds and then exhale. This type of breathing is used by first responders, military and athletes. It is used in elite training and allows you to stay focused in high stress situations. It is proven to lower blood pressure, release stress and tension, and even positively affects your heart and organs.

With your eyes open and focused, your breathing commenced, know that you will soon notice your eyes become heavy as you count backwards to yourself from 5 down to 1. Your eyes will become tired from the stare and will desire to close. Don't fight the urge, roll with it.

On 5 – Invite your creative imagination to take part in the process. Release from the need to overanalyze the process.

On 4 – As if you're entering into a space between now and tomorrow; a powerful space in time where you can let go of all worries and cares. A space between where you can focus on the inside and melt into a deep trust within yourself.

On 3 – You may notice that your eyes begin to now feel heavy, droopy, relaxed.

On 2 – Blinking eyes, now want to close.

On 1 – Focus on the inside, allowing yourself to deeply connect with a quiet space within you.

You can be quiet even though your thoughts may wander. You can gently bring your thoughts back into focus—on your heartspace and your breathing. Turning down the volume of your head chatter is a learned practice.

Continue to breathe deeply. You are creating physiological changes in your brain and body. Any time your mind wanders into monkey mind, direct your awareness back to the slow, easy rhythms you are creating between your mind, breath and heart. Now deepen that experience.

Deepen the experience with what we refer to as progressive relaxation. Starting at the crown of your head, direct your awareness toward the relaxation of those muscles. Create ease by thinking of ease. Imagine, think, know or feel your muscles releasing tension and becoming loose, limp and relaxed.

Ask the *color of relaxation* to pop into your mind.

That color represents your subconscious association with relaxation. Trust it is the right one for you. Many people are often surprised at their color, as it's not the one they would consciously choose, but it's been chosen for them by their subconscious.

Imagine, visualize and think about that color as if it is mobile and fluid. Let it flow with ease throughout your head and slowly down your neck and shoulders. Continue natural deep breaths all the while.

Progressively move the color like a wave of ease and

relaxation down the arms into the fingers, down the chest and particularly giving attention to the spine—seeing, visualizing or feeling as if the color is moving down each vertebra. Within each vertebra is rejuvenation and ease. Imagine yourself loose, limp and wonderfully flexible.

Your spine represents support. Breathe beautiful affirmative thoughts of gratitude towards your spine as it has supported you all through life. Send thoughts of healing and wholeness to your spine. This is particularly beneficial as many of us have beaten our bodies up with cruel language or dissatisfied thoughts. Use this time to experience a new gratitude for your body.

Move your color, that special color, down into your hips and abdomen. Imagine, visualize and think about your hips in a healing and restful state.

Like a wave of soothing, peaceful relaxation, send your color down your legs, giving special attention to the knees, reminding your knees of how wonderfully flexible they are. Send thoughts of gratitude to your knees for all the flexing and bending they do. Send affirmative thoughts of healing to the knees as if to lubricate the knees with your beautiful color.

Send your color down into your calves, shins and ankles. Imagine, visualize and think about your color easing its way down into your feet and that vivid color of special relaxation oozing into the heels, arches and balls of your feet. Once again, send gratitude into your feet. After all, they've taken you far. Appreciate them for a moment. Think, feel and say, "Thank you."

It is in this state of calm, clarity and focus that you can explore, detach and release psychological and emotional attachments. Release grievances and invite in miracles. Utilize this special time as if you are planting a garden. You can cultivate your thoughts, just as you cultivate a garden. Pull weeds, plant new seeds. Think of it as a beautiful, organic process, as in nature, of seeding, cultivating and harvesting. Soon you will harvest a new result in your body.

Throughout this book you are asked to journal and express your thoughts through F.I.T. Exercises. Use the F.I.T. Method process shared here as your method to engaging with the questions and exercises throughout. As you learned earlier in this chapter, this method engages your alpha and theta brain waves where science has proven a higher state of focus and openness. It is ideal to interact from this state as it is a fast and effective process for change. You will not be using your analytical mind, but instead, your powerful subconscious. Yay! A new approach to your goals is refreshing. This process is a particularly powerful way to shed pounds as it is not focused on an external diet, but instead, focused on how you feed your mind. Sure, eating habits and exercise will play a part. But we want to approach those things from a new perspective.

While using this technique throughout the book, count yourself down from 5 to 1. Then open your eyes to journal your answers. With practice, you'll deepen your process and you'll soon love how easy it is. You may notice a shift in your physical presence as a result of the exercise. That's perfectly normal. Some report a tingling, others feel deeply relaxed muscles, and even a stirring of their emotions. When prompted, ask the respective question to yourself while in the deep relaxed state. Your awareness will bring up answers and insights. Then open your eyes and journal away.

After you journal your answers, be sure to count yourself back up with the following sequence.

On 1 – Slowly, calming and with ease, awakening fully.

On 2 – Calibrating all levels of consciousness—mental, physical, emotional, cellular, spiritual.

On 3 – Alive and refreshed.

On 4 – As if you've bathed your eyes in cool, fresh, spring water.

On 5 – Wide awake, clear, confident and ready.

You can also use this method to practice relieving stress and anxiety at any time. You can center yourself before a big moment like a speaking opportunity, test or interview. You can use it to fall asleep faster or as a 5-minute power nap in your work day. I'll be sharing with you throughout the chapters many exercises that can greatly improve your well-being and performance. It is suggested that you practice the F.I.T. Method and integrate it into your life as a tool to assist your personal growth in all manners. Get accustomed to using it often!

Short Format to Easily Reference the Process

1 – Place your hand on your heart for calibration.

2 – Fixate your eyes.

3 – Incorporate deep breathing.

4 – Count backwards 5-1 using creative thoughts to deepen, slowly closing your eyes when ready.

5 – Deepen to another level using progressive relaxation and color creativity.

6 – Insert soul question, affirmations or a visualization.

7 – Count yourself back up 1-5.

Get excited! You're about to begin your journey. In the next chapter, we'll dive into your desires. My goal is to start you off with building a deep foundation as to why you are making the effort to take care of yourself better. The insights I share will beckon you to look within and discover new reasons for living a health-optimized life of energy and vitality. With your new F.I.T. Method Superpower, you can do anything!

I invite you to visit my website at DeAnnaNunez.com to experience a F.I.T. Session in which I personally guide you on video.

Chapter 2

Decide You Matter

The starting point of great success and achievement has always been the same. It is for you to dream big dreams.
~ Brian Tracy

Heavy Exhalation ...
Constant attention to my eating habits is so much work. It's much easier to just get over it and live with the fact that I'm heavier than I use to be. I don't care so much about six pack abs. But dang it, at the same time, it's just so frustrating because I do want to look and feel my best.

Most definitely, you are due for a fresh perspective. It's important to remember why you have chosen this journey to living healthy. It is definitely a choice. At times it may seem much easier to go back to your old way of doing things; less work and fewer personal commitments, but just because it becomes difficult doesn't mean you should give up on your goal of having a fit, lean body. Let me remind you of why you would want to stick with creating this new lifestyle. **It's because YOU matter.**

MAKE THE DECISION TO BE WHAT IT TAKES

Imagine visiting the park for a day of picnicking and relaxing in the warm afternoon sun. After parking the car, you follow a winding dirt trail through a dry, rocky landscape knowing there must be lush ground ahead. The search is on for the perfect scenic spot. As you venture down the trail you are greeted with a flourishing canyon of picturesque rock and wildflowers. From where you stand, the surroundings are rugged, yet just across the canyon are blooming hillsides, and tall swaying trees. As you gaze across the gorge you notice a flat, grassy area alongside the river's edge. It's the perfect lunching spot. Your eyes begin to scout for a bridge or rocks to traverse the river. With excitement to get to the other side, you think, *there must be a way.* And with determination you set off to find a crossing.

The gap between the harsh, unforgiving land and the inviting picnic spot is where the true journey lies. You must navigate your way to cross over from the years of battling your body to a lifestyle of loving your body and nurturing it. The opportunity is before you, and it matters that you cross the rocks to the other side. All you have to do is make the decision. Decide that however difficult the passage may be, the trip will be worth your efforts. Your picnic will be that much more enjoyable because of the fact that it is in a location that is less traveled, a place you can call your own secret sanctuary. It's about who you become as a result of your effort.

To enjoy the best life possible, you must consider your fitness health. Your dreams, aspirations and relationships are all compromised if you don't. This includes your emotional and mental health as well. In an article published by *Scientific American,* it is noted that vigorous physical exercise is critical to mental health. So, although fitting into skinny jeans may be an awesome feeling and a target to shoot for, it's not just about aesthetics. There must be a deeper reason.

F.I.T. QUESTION

What is the pain of not taking this health journey?

- Place your hand on your heart for calibration.

- Fixate your eyes.

- Breathe deeply – inhale 4 seconds,
  pause 4 seconds, exhale 4 seconds.

- Count backwards 5-1 using creative thoughts to
  deepen, slowly closing your eyes when ready.

- Deepen to another level using progressive
  relaxation and your special color.

- Insert the question above. Then, open
  your eyes and journal the question.

- Close your eyes back down and count
  yourself up 1-5, opening your eyes on 5.

UNTRUE TRUTHS MESS WITH YOUR HEAD

There are women who use their bodies as a means to hide. They have learned to believe they are incapable of enjoying certain experiences in life because of their body. The Joie de Vivre—a French phrase for the "Joys of Life"—may not be fully expressed simply because they live in a body they have not embraced.

Some women I speak with are so unhappy with their bodies that they stop having sex. They don't think they are as sexy as they once were and feel uncomfortable being naked. They are insecure with their bodies and make up beliefs about what their partners think of them. Often those beliefs are unfounded, yet they allow their own feelings about their body to skew their judgment, and a communication breakdown drives a wedge between the couple. If you've been a culprit in this limiting belief, you've done both your partner and you a colossal disservice. If you've had a partner who expressed words of dislike or disdain about your body, it may be time to have a mature communicative talk. Because that's not okay.

The single ladies can also fall in a mind trap with sex. Have you stopped putting yourself out there? Consensual, healthy sex is a part of overall optimal health and sexuality. Whether you are single or with a long-time partner I encourage you to open-up. Explore. Invite in intimacy. Get out of your head and experience the alpha states of consciousness that healthy sexuality delivers. And if there is something that needs to be healed or addressed in order to do so, be brave and do the growth work.

How can I be more open? Is there something I need to let go of to do so?

_____

_____

_____

_____

_____

Having experienced a sexual assault at just 15 years old, I know the impact it had on my mind and body for many years thereafter. Roughly 60% of the women who have gone through my programs have had some type of sexual abuse. It is often the hidden subconscious trauma that makes it very difficult for women to stay consistent with health routines. Other women simply stop being as active once they've gained weight or gotten older. They forget what it was like to feel young and full of energy. The old bike collects spider webs in the garage, and the treadmill becomes a dumping ground for the ironing. Even middle-aged moms cease playing with their children in a physical way and limit themselves just to the non-moving activities—books, cooking and crafts. They let dad do the physical stuff.

I once took my two children to a park while on a business trip in Ohio. When we arrived at the playground, I observed a group of moms sitting on the park bench. Some were engaging in conversation while eating fast food, others were on their phones while their kids played on the equipment. I went on with my purpose for visiting the park and started a game of tag the tree with my kids. Before long we had all the other children playing with us too. We had about a dozen kids running from tree to tree, counting off as they tagged the tree, and running to the next one. It was fun; I got my exercise and they did too! I probably burned off the amount of calories that the moms on the bench had consumed.

The only difference between those moms and me is, I have a different mindset. The moms overlooked their options while at the park. They could have gotten off the bench; smiled, laughed and played with their kids, but they didn't exercise their opportunity. Imagine how much fun the kids would have had with mom. Think about the opportunity she could have given them to live by example?

"I'm tired" is one of those mindset things you are making true. But it's not always true. Some days you just don't want to make the effort, or straight up legit, you're out of shape and making the effort feels tiring. Okay, ouch! I know that was a bit straightforward, but I promised to tell you the truth. You're here to do something about it and make the days of your life matter.

There are those gals, and perhaps you're one of them, who is driven, striving for your goals despite having struggled with your body. Our Mind Body F.I.T. community friend Genelle has said, "Weight becomes the big elephant in the room." Conquering goals, making the deadlines and achieving success, yet doing so with a lack of achievement in one major area of life—your health. Whatever your deal is, your body and health challenges are affecting your performance in life. Your HEALTH matters because YOU matter.

The real deal, and the reason I am reaching out to you through the work that I do, is I believe you have the right to live in the healthiest, most beautiful body for you. I also believe with the strongest conviction that your body is an interpretation of what's going on in your head. You are what your subconscious believes you are.

F.I.T. QUESTION

What have you been holding on to that you can now let go of?

- Place your hand on your heart for calibration.

- Fixate your eyes.

- Breathe deeply—inhale 4 seconds, pause 4 seconds, exhale 4 seconds.

- Count backwards 5-1 using creative thoughts to deepen, slowly closing your eyes when ready.

- Deepen to another level using progressive relaxation and your special color.

- Ask yourself: What have you been holding on to that you can now let go of?

_____

_____

_____

_____

_____

_____

_____

_____

Open your eyes and journal the question on paper.

- Close your eyes back down and count yourself up 1-5, opening your eyes on 5.

YOUR LIFE WILL MIRROR YOUR BELIEFS

Raised by a single mom, forever bitter by her divorce, I grew up with a strong sense of anger in my daily environment. Dad was attentive and loving, but I only spent time with him every other weekend. Mom made it very difficult for him to be more involved. The gaps that weren't being filled felt like the Grand Canyon. Like vast spaces of loneliness. I could often just fall into the abyss of worthlessness.

Between the ages of 13 to 18, I ran away repeatedly, shoplifted, stole family members' cars, drank to get drunk, smoked cocaine, was sexually assaulted and dropped out of school. I'm sure I've left a few things out, and rightly so, because telling you this is not for the purpose of hype or poor-me's, but to convey to you that I know the depths of despair, anguish and self-sabotage. In that timeframe, I actually attracted a really great boyfriend that genuinely cared for me, but I found a way to mess that up too. The only way for me to navigate those deep dark crevices that lived inside of me was to armor up and pretend that I didn't give a shit.

As you can imagine, the things I was doing scared the heck out of Mom. She had lived a sheltered, good-girl life. She was a churchgoer, a loyal wife and daughter, and judgmental of all things outside of her tunnel vision. So, when I began rebelling, she was not prepared to handle the adversity. Her reaction to my rebelliousness was to label me. I can recall the exact spot I was in when it happened. My old bedroom downstairs. I was standing next to my massive oak waterbed. Mom and

I were having a huge fight. Her eyes pooled with tears, her face harsh with criticism and her finger pointing at me with disgust as she spouted,

"You are never going to amount to anything!"

BOOM! There it is. Shot through the heart with shame and worthlessness. That one line stuck with me like it was a life sentence.

I had already felt like the biggest loser on the planet and that statement sealed the deal. After those formidable years, I lived my life thinking and doing things from a mediocre existence. Although I spent much of my alone time dreaming about a life of grandeur, my reality was nothing of the sort. After all, my unconscious believed I would never amount to much anyway. Thankfully I was no longer repeating the patterns of my teenager years, but I was just stuck, feeling uninspired by school, relationships or career.

You may have found yourself in a similar experience where something was said by someone you cared about, and it stuck with you negatively. As if the words of another deflated your balloon. As a result, you put yourself out there less often for fear of getting hurt or noticed. When you play small, people have little to say. For those that have experienced abuse, it's a tactic that keeps you safe.

Trauma can also spur the competitive edge. Being driven can make you so focused on succeeding that you will do anything it takes to overcome the emotional pain that still plays in the back of your head. Sometimes people charge their way through life with the need to prove their worth. This method can be devastating as your internal cry keeps you from true connection and steals your ability to be peaceful within. Never truly satisfied.

I've also seen it with women ambitious for a cause or an entrepreneurial goal. The trauma of their childhood or past keeps them so focused on changing others' lives, they ignore internally changing their own. There is a dark void that continually gets filled by serving others, but it's like a boat with a hole in the bottom. They have to keep up the high pace of service to stay on top of the pain. Meanwhile their body is suffering by holding on to the weight of that unresolved conflict and their boat is slowly sinking.

One of my favorite mentors, Dr. David Hawkins says, "People that are hurting either project, suppress or repress." To project is to blame people or outside circumstances for our pain. To suppress is to numb ourselves with distractions or vices to avoid feeling the pain. And to repress is to push the pain so deep down inside that you go into denial about your hidden truth, smiling as if nothing is wrong. Our gift, as evolved women, is to know ourselves so deeply and truly that we have the power to heal ourselves and the world.

I know what it's like to be in the darkness of unworthiness. I also know what it's like to stand in front of 10,000 people speaking, performing and having so much fun living what feels like a dream. Over the years I have performed for governors, five star generals, opened for top musical acts, performed on cruise ships and for Fortune 500 companies.

I have stood in moments that I once dreamt about as a little girl. I knew by the age of eight that I wanted to be on stage. I could visualize myself up there smiling and dancing in a big way. In fact, I had a vision. The funny thing is I have an off-key singing voice and never did take a dance class or acting class, so what was I thinking? Good thing hypnosis came along. Even still, for years I let my negative experiences hinder my dreams and skew my worthiness. That message of, *You'll never amount to anything,* haunted me for decades. It also pushed me to prove it wrong. No matter how much clout my career provided, I still could not drown out the sound of Mom's voice and that awful mantra. I was hustling for my worthiness.

It would be years later that I learned to communicate with my subconscious and reframe. Reframing is a process we use in psychology and coaching to help our clients breakthrough mental barriers. I used it on myself to reframe my mother's paralyzing statement, and I found my worth again. I used the F.I.T. Method to bypass critical thinking, get underneath the raw emotion and forgive my mother.

Here's how I did it. I used the power of *visualization* combined with *auditory* and *linguistic* strength. I'd focus on a target point, count myself down, breathe and close my eyes. I call it getting connected. I then imagined her calm and still with her hands open and accepting. I visualized her that way as if she was standing right in front of me. I pictured and heard her saying the words, "You amount to everything."

I started to mantra her words from, "You'll never

amount to anything," to "You amount to everything." I did it repeatedly day after day. To provoke change at a subconscious level you must have two factors—repetition and emotion. This practice completely dissolved the emotional charge and I was able to create my own breakthrough. Now, it's your turn.

JOURNAL F.I.T. QUESTION

Did you have any negative experiences like that? Perhaps with a parent, an ex-husband, a teacher, colleague, sibling or a group of kids? Something that was said that stuck with you for years and you measured yourself by it?

Write out the words here:

_____

_____

_____

_____

_____

_____

Reframe them to a positive statement here:

_____

_____

_____

_____

Now use the F.I.T. Method to internalize your new framing.

- Place your hand on your heart for calibration.

- Fixate your eyes.

- Deep breathing.

- Count backwards 5-1 using creative thoughts to deepen, slowly closing your eyes when ready.

- Deepen to another level using progressive relaxation and your special color.

- Insert reframing here.

- Count yourself back up 1-5.

WHERE THERE IS LOVE, THERE IS HEALING

The difference between self-worth and self-confidence is an important distinction. Self-confidence is based on competence in a specific skill set(s). Whereas self-worth is the sum of the value you feel you bring to the world. It considers the idea that your very existence has meaning. That the world would truly be missing something valuable if you weren't here to contribute.

You can very well have a strong self-worth, yet lack self-confidence in a particular area. For instance, if you are a person who has attempted a health-behavior change (diet, restricted foods, exercise regimen) and failed multiple times, your self-confidence in knowing how to manage your healthiest weight has been depleted. That does not mean you don't value yourself or are lacking in self worth. Yet, I've seen many women make one mean the other.

Your self-worth, according to a research study called the Contingencies of Self-Worth Scale (developed by researchers Crocker, Luhtanen, Cooper and Bouvrette 2003) is derived from a balance of seven specific aspects that include achievements and/or performance, significant relationships you cultivate with family love and support, being a moral person, approval from self and others, physical appearance, academic competence and spiritual connection.

In my work, I've observed some of us lean into one area more than another based on the significance of our own life experiences. Perhaps you had a parent that put a strong emphasis on academic achievement, therefore it is how you unconsciously measure your self-worth. Or, an environment or culture that measured self-worth from beauty. To a degree, all these things carry their own bias. It is your opportunity to make decisions for yourself on how you can better balance these attributes and draw out the untruths that may be attached. Mark Twain said, "A man cannot be comfortable without his own approval." Perhaps its time to start approving of yourself.

When you distill it all down, it is unarguable that it is no accident you are here. Your birth was on purpose. No matter what circumstances created that, your presence, your soul, the contribution of your own uniqueness is here to add something beautiful to the world. As you allow yourself to internalize that truth, imagine the feeling of fulfillment you can create in your life. My feeling is that we can unite self-worth and self-confidence into a new hybrid model. I like how Brendon Burchard describes self-confidence. His take is that *it's the ability to know you'll figure things out.* That puts the responsibility of your life results back on you.

As a woman with a desire to design your mind, life and body, it is your gift to yourself to take full ownership of that. Stop questioning your worth. You are worth what you are because you are. End of discussion. Let's proceed with that assumption. After all, your subconscious mind responds to what you believe. Within this book, my intention is to build your fitness upon a foundation of both self-worth and self-confidence. You'll learn to bring your sense of self value into your thinking habits, and I'll bring you important aspects to consider in terms of attaching that to daily actions of self-care.

HOW HAS YOUR LIFE HELPED MOLD YOU?

To be fit now, it's important that you consider what brought you to this place, reading this book. You may be here because you're looking for solutions. That's great. It tells me you're on a path for change. So often when we desire change, our first choice is to leave the past behind. Although it is a fruitful decision to move forward, I'd like you to consider how your past has delivered important lessons that are greatly valuable to your present life.

I was a divorced, single mother at 21 years old. My adorable son Zach became my saving grace. The word birth is defined as starting new. His very presence did that for me. The unconditional love I felt through him made me want to be a better person. Although I was relatively lost and operating off of very low self-confidence, I felt the glimmer of hope lighting up inside me. I wanted success for the two of us. In search of a life I could be proud of, I began looking for ways to be more positively influenced. Wayne Dyer says, "We don't get what we want, we get what we intend." Intention comes from a deep, spiritual force within you and when you direct it for your good, its power draws people and opportunities to fulfill your intention. Intend for your life to be successful.

From the spirit of intention I was introduced to a man who would unintentionally show me a way to change my life. Later in the book, we'll discuss the importance of these mentors and how to recognize them. This man was an unlikely mentor to me, even though at the time, he seemed nothing of the sort. He was a man I got set up with on a blind date. A friend called one day and said she wanted to set me up with her boyfriend's cousin. I rolled my eyes and asked, as any woman does, "Well, what's he like?" She answered, "He's kinda short, balding, and hairy, but he's really funny!" I thought, *hardly my dark and handsome type,* but the funny part intrigued me.

As it turned out, he was a Comedy Stage Hypnotist and he seemed to have his finger on the pulse of his success. Within just months of dating and hanging out at his performances, one night his stage assistant abruptly quit the show. She had played the part of 'Vanna White of Hypnosis'; assisting the Hypnotist with sound cues, props, and looking pretty in her dazzling dress of the evening. Next thing I know, I am being cleverly persuaded into her position. I willingly accepted the opportunity with the idea that it would be exciting to travel, have more laughs, and live a lifestyle that seemed full of fun. Yet, I'm a single mom. My little Zach would need to go to his dad's when I'm out doing shows. We worked it out and I proceeded to make something of this new opportunity.

To be on stage. Yikes! Part of me wanted to be that girl, but another part did not feel worthy of such a status. I felt like the audience would see right through my facade. I could be up on stage acting confident, pretending, but it was truly just an act. I was severely self-conscious of my weight, and felt that everyone in the audience was picking me apart. Have you ever played that role in your head? It's a form of imposter syndrome. I know you probably have and you can relate to my insecurities.

I could stand up there on stage playing the part, but when it came to speaking in front of the audience, that was another playing field. I had little confidence, and the belief that I had nothing significant to say. Night after night, as part of my duties, I had to announce the Star Hypnotist as he came on to the stage. I wanted to die every time. In fact, I know you know the statistics—more people would rather die than speak publicly. Yep, I was in that category. Maybe you are too? I would actually hide in order to get the job done. I was the invisible voice behind the curtain.

After two years together, and literally hundreds of shows around the world, we parted ways. That part of the story was also meant to be. He went on to meet the love of his life, and so did I. But after we went our separate directions, I found myself contemplating with a friend on what I should do for a job. I questioned my future. Should I go back to what I was doing before my whirlwind hypnosis experience? Makeup artistry and cosmetology had been my field of choice, but somehow it seemed dull in comparison.

From that relationship, I have many adventurous and fun memories. I also gained tremendous stage experience, and valuable insight into the World of Hypnosis. Little did I realize, that boyfriend had given me more than just an opportunity to travel, he led me to a future career, and a path to truly making a difference in the world. That entire experience also set me up to truly get a handle on my mindset around my weight. Little did I know, it would soon all unfold in my favor.

JOURNAL F.I.T. QUESTION

What unexpected experience have you had that ended up delivering you to a new place in your life? And how can you use that valuable learning now to create confidence in your journey moving forward?

BLASTING THROUGH MENTAL BLOCKS

In my work as a Hypnotist, I've learned how to reveal, release and recode a mental block. It's become my signature process. You most likely have a mental block that is keeping you from your ideal weight. It is an irrational belief that you keep in your subconscious, and although it hinders your success, you unconsciously believe it's protecting you, therefore it sticks around. I thought I needed to be a size six to get on stage to perform an Edutainment Hypnosis Show. I didn't think people would want to look at a chunky girl with a microphone. *I need to get skinny. I need to be good on my diet.* Those were the constant words swirling the back of my head. It was a major mental block!

I continued to peel back the layers with hypnosis sessions, and I realized I was using my extra body fat as an excuse to never truly achieve my goals. It was my way of staying unhappily comfortable; my way of having a reason as to why I couldn't pursue more in my life. I was taking the back seat and letting my old, mediocre thinking lead the way. Every schoolteacher I had in high school would say, "She's just not living up to her potential." I was used to not fully engaging in my abilities. After all, Mom said I'd never amount to much. So I didn't try very hard. I was clearly underestimating myself.

I intuitively knew that to be successful on stage I had to go do it. There was no room for toying with the idea. I had performed so many shows with my previous experience, and I was growing quite tired of sabotaging myself. It was now or never. I needed to trust my instinct, and flail myself out there. This is the part of the hero's journey where a life of adventure or a greater calling shouts your name. With a greater vision, I performed my very first show on my own. It was terrifying and exhilarating at the same time. In the car, on the way home from the gig, I said with relief, *I never have to do my first presentation again. It's all good from here on out.* Performing that show in a body I didn't love, risking the embarrassment and doing it anyway was the first time I felt truly empowered. The day after that show was the first day of the rest of my life as a self-assured woman. It didn't happen all at once, but as a gradual process to uncovering the real me.

After the first season of traveling on the road performing, I returned to California five months later and several sizes smaller. I had shed weight naturally by actively being courageous and changing my thinking habits. With each performance I stepped out of my comfort zone time and time again and leaped beyond the old self-esteem issues. That leap paid off! Thank goodness I took a chance on myself. I later married the love of my life, and we have been together for over twenty years now.

He and I met back in those first days of going through hypnotherapy training. He loved me as the chunky girl with the false confidence and has watched me grow into a whole woman. He has stuck around as I've climbed mountains and sailed deep oceans of self-doubt. Together we developed, produced and performed hypnosis presentations all over the United States and overseas. Miraculously, the extra body weight that I had been gaining and losing for so many years came off without dieting.

For the very first time, I wasn't even trying to lose weight. I was simply standing in my own power. Owning my power meant that I cared what I ate, and that I prioritize my time to include exercise. It was a psychological shift from desperation to empowerment. So here's the thing. When you fully stand in your power, you love who you are. When you love who you are, you tend to make better eating choices and stay more active. Blasting through your mental blocks is not just mental. Your mind and body are connected.

JOURNAL F.I.T. EXERCISE

Place your hand on your heart. Focus your eyes. Inhale and exhale three to five deep breaths. Close and deepen. Do this between each soul question. Listen for the answers and then journal.

In what way have you taken a back seat to your true potential?

_____

_____

_____

_____

In what ways have you used your body as an excuse to not do something?

_____

_____

_____

_____

In what way can you reframe your thinking, forgive yourself and move forward?

_____

_____

_____

_____

YOUR SIGNIFICANCE

Do you feel significant to the world? Do you feel like you matter to the people around you? These are important questions to ask yourself, but the answer is not an external one. The answer must come from within you. You cannot measure your significance by what others think, say or even credit you with. You have to care about yourself enough to get your butt off the couch. That's step one. Despite overscheduling, and a multitude of priorities, it's your responsibility to show yourself that you care enough about you to make living healthy a significant part of your life.

You, and only you, are responsible for etching out a life that you can feel good about. Your significance in the world can only be truly measured by the greatness you allow within. When you know you've done the things you said you would do, when you've been the example of what you'd want your kids to be, and when you've struggled and persevered, then you can feel peace within knowing that your life matters. To do this, you've got to reach for what you want.

As much as a mom wants her baby to walk, she can't do it for her. I can remember being on the floor with my little one saying, "Come on, you can do it," as she struggled to make all her limbs move harmoniously together. She'd flop on her belly, take an accidental nosedive towards the carpet or roll over. It was most definitely a feat she was tenacious to figure out. Her determination was innate. She didn't sit around thinking, *Oh I can't because of this or that,* she just kept at it until she completed the task; each time learning a little more of what to do and what not to do. I could help by holding out my fingers, encourage her with my words, but the act of walking had to be done all on her own.

This health journey is an act you must figure out. You've spent way too much time feeling bamboozled, lost and defeated or plain old ignoring it altogether. Now is your time to bring forth the realization that the choices you make, and how you take care of your health, is significant in your world.

Your life matters. How you spend your time and the impact you choose to make in your life, makes a difference. You may have unique talents that are untapped and dormant. I believe hiding your personal gifts is a disfavor to your life. Would you advise a budding young woman to NOT use her talents; hindering her growth and personal development? Of course you wouldn't! Imagine having wonderful gifts wrapped up beautifully under the Christmas tree and never opening them. I encourage you to take off the wrapping, expose the gift inside and put it to good use! You may very well have strengths and abilities that, perhaps you never realized, would be so useful to your health journey.

Perhaps you are a great cook. If you learned to transform your favorite dishes into healthy delicious meals, you could be an asset to your friends, neighbors and family that are struggling to eat right. Heck, you could even be the next healthy cooking star on the Food Network. Maybe you are a natural leader, but you are leading your friends in an unbeneficial direction getting together for Martini Night, rather than a brisk walk around the neighborhood or a weekend hike. You could utilize your leadership skills to rally your friends in joining you for an accountability get-together once a week, or even lead your friends in training for a women's 10K to support a good cause.

The time is now for a mind awakening. Every woman in the universe has some unique quality that can be the missing piece to her healthy body puzzle. The only way to discover your inner resources is to interact with your feelings, thoughts and aspirations. It's time to dream again!

This healthy, mind-body journey that you take with me will be from a much different perspective than what you've grown accustomed to with dieting in the past. I'm going to ask you to discover your passion for life and use it as a catalyst to help you conquer your struggle with weight. If you don't know what you're passionate about, that's great too. I guarantee this process will help you to get closely connected with your insides so that your outside becomes a new reflection of YOU. Soon you could be living a life free from stressing about fitting into your clothes, free from talking about what diet you're on (that you call a lifestyle) and free from worrying about gaining weight at the holidays no longer loving yourself with food or using food as your favorite pastime saying, "I don't know why, I just love to eat!"

Along my journey to becoming fit, I learned that food will never feed me like self-worth will. I have taken care of the emotional eating behaviors that once imprisoned me and adopted a new mindset. I still have challenges, we all do. It's called Life. Yet I feel equipped to overcome those challenges by practicing the strategies that I share with you in this book, beginning with the F.I.T. Strategy next.

My hope is for you to discover your own *OMG moments* (Oh My Gosh, I can't believe I have been doing that to myself). Trust that you have this information in your hands because it is the right time. I ask that you accept the challenge to get honest with yourself and have the courage to uncover what you have possibly stuffed down inside. I discovered that I'm worth the effort it takes to better myself. I know you're worth it too. Are you ready to discover the body and life of your dreams? Are you ready to believe in yourself? It's never too late.

In the next chapter, you'll learn the attitude that will explosively start your journey to getting the results you want. Be willing to open your mind to new ideas and perceptions. Let's go friend! Jump with me in a leap of faith.

MANTRA
"I matter in the world."

F.I.T. STRATEGY EXERCISE
Because I Matter

- Sit down with paper and pen.
  Use the F.I.T. Method.

- The reflection question is, *what is important about my presence in the world?*

- Place your hand on your heart for calibration.

- Fixate your eyes.

- Deep breathing.

- Count backwards 5-1 using creative thoughts to deepen, slowly closing your eyes when ready.

- Deepen to another level using progressive relaxation and color therapy.

- What is important about my presence in the world? Ask yourself this question and notice what bubbles up. Open your eyes and journal.

- Count yourself back up 1-5.

_____

_____

_____

_____

_____

Chapter 3

Up Your Willingness Game

No one is in control of your happiness but you, therefore, you have the power to change anything about yourself or your life that you want to change.

~ Barbara de Angelis

Willingness is a cheerful agreement you make with yourself. When you are willing, you are in a state of continuous flowing growth. It is nonjudgmental and an ever-evolving state of mind. You are free of reluctance. You are optimistic, excited about the possibilities of the future and eager to learn.

Willingness is readiness; showing up to your life and being ready for anything that comes your way. You have to be willing to do what other people are not, in order to achieve health success. You have to be willing to take the necessary steps to overcome any obstacle that enters your path. That is true willingness.

I ask you ... What are you willing to change in order to have a fit, lean body? What are you willing to sacrifice?

Perhaps you're thinking, *Whoooaaa! Wait a minute De'Anna, that's all too much!* And you are right. It is too much all at once. Let me lift your worries. All you really have to do at this point in the process is be willing to believe there is a way to your health goal outside of strict dieting.

To open up your willingness, I invite you to explore your unwillingness. Many times a woman with a closed mind doesn't even recognize herself to be this way. Perhaps she is a volunteer for her daughter's Brownie Troop or a leader amongst her peers in her industry. She is visibly present in activities, but when it comes to her personal health, she's closed off. The woman with a closed mind is rigid and inflexible; no longer receiving, or growing. She builds emotional walls and chooses to live life disconnected from herself; as if she can remain anonymous there. Her walls act as a shield, protecting her from that in which she is not ready to manage. Within this lonely existence it's as if she remains fragile and broken, just wanting to be accepted and loved. She may say she wants to get healthy but is unwilling to face her fears and insecurities. The most disappointing aspect of a woman unwilling to believe in herself is that she doesn't have to be this way. It truly comes down to the fundamental need for unconditional love. No matter your stature or position in life, not one of us is exempt from it. We all seek love and acceptance.

I once guided a hypnosis session wherein my client was a very powerful CEO. The ability to achieve great financial success was a focus she conquered having made millions of dollars in her career. Unbeknownst to the outside world, she felt alone and unloved on the inside. Our session revealed a childhood of abandonment and fear. Although as an adult she had obtained what many strive for in life, she still felt incomplete. Great financial success was the one thing that temporarily filled that void. It was her way of proving herself worthy. Obtaining success gave her fulfillment, but it became exhausting trying to keep up the charade. What she was truly after was love.

While you read through these pages, I am asking you to be willing to delve into the process of discovering your unconditional self-love. The distance between where you are now and where you imagine yourself to be in your ideal healthy body starts with a willing attitude to show yourself love. As you embark on this journey, you'll find that inspiration is all around you. By reaching out and being willing to admit that you could use some guidance, you will create an energy shift in the way that you shine in the world. All that you need to guide you will show up in your life.

In the following pages, my clients share their stories, journeys and self-care tips.

STARR'S STORY

Willingness

As I was doing the research to write about willingness, I turned to one of my favorite resources: the online dictionary. This definition popped up: "Eagerly Compliant." I laughed at that definition, because I knew that when I first started my health journey, "eagerly compliant" wasn't something I felt. I had a desire to be healthy, however, I didn't possess the willingness to move into action. Back then I was allowing fear to trump the love I didn't realize I had for myself.

My transformation started nine years ago, and it has taken all these years to become willing to allow health, happiness and love into my life. I reflect on the choices I've made to become who I am right now in this moment. I am a woman who's choosing to stand in her power. I've released almost 90 pounds and I am taking control of my health, despite kidney disease and multiple life struggles. To leave the weight behind, I had to leave lots of other things, too. I chose to leave my second marriage that was entrapped with physical and emotional abuse. I left friends, ideas and family members. I left behind a beautiful home and community for homelessness. I left it all behind to float on the river of willingness to love myself.

The Shift

I can recall the exact moment my heart became willing. I was 1,200 miles away from my kids and while on the phone with my husband, he told me that in a moment of anger he had dumped cereal on our daughter's head. That act was so utterly unacceptable to me. I would do anything in my power to not repeat patterns from my childhood. It was in that moment willingness for growth and change went from desire to mental action. It was the circumstance outside of me that propelled my willingness for change. Perhaps for you it doesn't have to be that blatant. I just happen to be a stubborn one. Today, I realize that it didn't have to take that experience in my life to make me be willing to do something about my health and our situation. My heart knew the truth. I knew the home my children and I were in was unhealthy, and not just because of my future ex-husband either. I had to look at myself more than ever. I was allowing this life. Many times, I had been prompted by my heart to heal my situation, to reach out, to find a way into a better feeling life. Finally I answered the call.

I asked myself this important question, "What is it that you do want and why?" I proclaimed it! I was willing to give up everything just to listen to that side of myself that said, "You deserve to love yourself." I just knew I didn't want to be labeled as unhealthy anymore. I am the girl who loves basketball, the girl who wants to learn how to play sports and ride a horse, the girl with an adventurous spirit to absorb every new thing I possibly can. I see myself as a fit and healthy girl. It was in my growth into womanhood that I'd lost that mindset. Somewhere along the way I stopped absorbing and learning from the world around me.

I became eager for my transformation because I found worthiness in who I am. I started to believe the vision within, and I was willing to allow that vision to guide me. I became willing to learn about the lack of worthiness that I felt inside. I started writing about my feelings of unworthiness and focusing inward. I focused my attention on topics that filled my mind and heart with value and worthiness. I started to address those feelings within me that felt difficult. I took what I learned and reshaped my mind. What used to look like a mountain in my mind now looked like a pebble. When I allowed ease to become a regular choice in my life, things started to shift, and the shift happened in a relatively short amount of time. The moment I said, "I am willing to follow Starr's own heart," was the moment momentum entered the playground of my life.

Divine Validation Steps In

One day I received a call from a friend and I was willing to hear the divinity. He said, "You're one of three people who has touched my life." In that phone call, I knew it was time. It was time to step into all that was there for me and know that the vision I had held onto for so many years was ready to be executed. I finally accepted who I am right where I am and that acceptance made my health journey that much more meaningful. Willingness began to feel like ease. Flow. Vibe. Willingness moved me from thought to action. I learned; all it takes is momentum to shift your mindset from one place to another. That momentum can create a habit knowing that what we practice we become.

We all have opportunities to allow willingness into our lives because deep down inside, willingness is just the reminder we need to be exactly who we are meant to be. When we follow our heart, it leads us to the beautiful places in our universe that allow us to see who we really are deep down inside. We give ourselves opportunities to prove who we are every single day. We can see ourselves as a canvas for growth, and then grow into who we see. It is then that we break through.

The winning in life is always because we choose it and practicing who we are on a daily basis will always be worth the effort.

MARCIA'S STORY

In the Mind Body F.I.T. community, we have a courageous woman whose name is Marcia. She's in her sixties and exemplifies this willingness trait to great extent. We have watched her transform into the most energetic, inspired fitness enthusiast South Carolina has ever seen.

She is involved in softball, bowling and religiously attends her favorite Zumba class. She is so pumped with exuberance that she even slides headfirst into home base during her softball games. Again, she's in her sixties! She is willing to lay it all on the line for her team. The motivation she has created comes from within and is attractive to all who know her. She even prides herself on how much dirt she comes home with on her jersey. Our Mind Body F.I.T. Club ladies now use the phrase "I Eat Dirt!" in honor of her contagious energy.

Her enthusiasm has not come from a life without toil. She has experienced her share of heartbreak and self-doubt. She was once in a bad first marriage and was repeatedly told that she was worthless and stupid. The memories of those years still create a feeling of sadness, knowing now that she had a choice. She's come a long way since those days. Through personal growth and healing, she now chooses to live her life inspired. She's even married to the man of her dreams who is supportive and loving.

This health journey is about acknowledging your whole self. You must adopt a willing approach to life; become a student who is ever-evolving. That may require you to be willing to risk feeling undesirable emotions, be willing to stand up for yourself or take a chance on letting people see the real you. This is not a weight loss competition or a before and after picture achieved by counting calories. It entails sifting through the old emotional crap that seems to be a recurring theme in your life. Your body has been holding on to all of it, like the junk drawer in your kitchen. Are you willing to sort through it?

We've all seen the TV shows that help families get rid of their junk. The experts come in to their unorganized existence and facilitate a transformation by quickly examining each item, then categorizing it into sections. They create three categories. Save. Trash. Give Away. After days of sifting through the years of piles and junk, the end result leaves the homeowner feeling uplifted and free to start a new life.

In this health journey process you will SAVE your talents, abilities, strengths, self esteem and confidence. TRASH the old excuses, pity parties, negative mindsets and beliefs. And GIVE AWAY the habits and junk foods that are not supporting your goals. In the end, you too will have an amazing feeling of freedom! Let's back up for moment. For this process to be successful ... you must start by being willing.

I believe, let me rephrase that, I know, that you are much more capable than you think you are. We have incorporated fitness events into our MBFC community as a regular practice, because participating in them builds personal confidence and belief. Walking or jogging your first 5 or 10K inspires you to believe in yourself. Not only do you prove to yourself that you CAN do it, but often, you prove that you could probably go even farther! You wouldn't have believed it, if you hadn't actually done it yourself.

You cannot get healthy through regimented tasks alone, you must engage your spirit; the deeper more powerful part of you. "The spirit indeed is willing, but the flesh is weak." This quote comes from biblical times, so you see this is not a new concept, but indeed a meaningful method for you to get healthy. A state of willingness empowers you to let go of all the old excuses. To overcome habituated patterns, Dr. Wayne Dyer said in his bestselling book *Excuses Be Gone,* "You'll ultimately realize that there are no excuses worth defending, ever, even if they've always been part of your life."

You may be creating excuses that seem legit, but they are not. There are a group of co-workers at a friend's company who get together to walk at lunchtime. They are varied shapes and sizes and mostly women. One of the heaviest women in the group creates constant conversation of how she wants to drop a few pounds, yet she often announces that once again she has forgotten her walking shoes at home. One of the other women finally told her to buy two pairs of shoes. One pair to keep at home, and another to keep at the office so that she wouldn't need to use that excuse anymore.

It's not entirely your fault that you may be overweight, out of shape or not your healthiest. Are you agreeing, shaking your head "yes" now? *Yeah, it's my job, it's so stressful, or I know it's not my fault, my husband eats crappy food and it's such a bad influence on me.* Uhhh ... girlfriend, wake up from that lie.

Your job is not the reason you are overweight. I won't apologize for being forward with you, because I know your mind is so powerful it can overcome anything with the right focus.

When I state that it's not your fault, I am referring to the power of the subconscious mind. In the next chapter we will explore deeper into your inner programming. But first make a commitment to yourself with this next F.I.T. Exercise to put all your excuses out on the table.

F.I.T. STRATEGY EXERCISE

Willingness

I am willing to commit to myself on a deeper level.

- Place your hand on your heart for calibration.

- Fixate your eyes.

- Deep breathing.

- Count backwards 5-1 using creative thoughts to deepen, slowly closing your eyes when ready.

- Deepen to another level using progressive relaxation and color therapy.

- Connect with the excuses and why you have them.

- Count yourself back up 1-5.

Write out the excuses you use to avoid eating better, exercising at your peak performance or as limiting factors to your success at shedding extra weight. Ask your inner mind to recall all the excuses you have allowed yourself to entertain. Write down the ludicrous ones, those that feel legitimate and why.

1 _____

_____

_____

_____

2 _____

_____

_____

_____

3 _____

_____

_____

_____

4 _____

_____

_____

_____

5 _____

_____

_____

_____

Great job being truthful with yourself! I am excited to share with you valuable insights in the next section. You will have a better understanding of why you do what you do, and how to overcome the limitations that are holding you back. Come with me ... I'll help you discover your courage.

Chapter 4

Know Thyself

*Nothing makes a woman more beautiful
than the belief that she is beautiful.*

~ Sophia Loren

You have been programmed by your life experiences. As a young child, you were very receptive and impressionable. You had not yet developed critical factoring, and therefore you simply took in information like a sponge. Anyone who had a direct influence in your life—parents, family members, teachers, pastors and others—constantly conveyed information that you collected unconsciously. It was during this period of early growth that your lifelong belief systems were developed, and behavioral patterns began to grow and mold based on those beliefs and inner identity. Situations, experiences, people and words made an impression on you. Even ways you live your life now is made up from all of that collective information.

Think about the word IMPRESSION and what it means. The dictionary describes it as: *a mark, or imprint. An effect produced, as on the mind or senses, by some force or influence.* You may very well be living with an imprint that does not align with who you want to be.

A Mind Body F.I.T. member shared that when she was a young girl, her mother took her to the Diet Center, a chain of weight loss centers in business in the 1980s. She walked from the car observing the sign on the building wondering why they were going there. Before she knew it, she was signed up and being told to eat a selection of their packaged foods. She recalls thinking that her mom felt the Diet Center would help her. Yet, she had been unaware there was a problem until then. This sent strong messages of inadequacy. She says she remembers thinking, *If I could be skinnier, my mom will love me more.*

This scenario truly exemplifies how the adults who reared us held great responsibility in influencing our belief systems. Our subconscious minds are shaped and molded by those who have had persuasive influence upon us as children. Every impressionable experience of your life, the ones with great emotional charge, leaves a mark or imprint within your subconscious mind. Those imprints cause that familiar voice in your head to speak positively or negatively to you.

Have you ever said:

I can't do it.

I've already blown it, I might as well eat the whole thing now.

I don't have time to exercise, I'm too busy.

Just this one brownie.

As I age, I keep gaining body weight.

Screw it, I'm fat anyway.

The list goes on and on, and so do the imprints. Many of those words in your head are not even your own. How many times have you said something, and as it falls out of your mouth, you realize you sound just like your mother, your father or ex-husband? Aha! You have an imprint.Your history can also influence you in positive ways, and perhaps you love that you have taken on certain characteristics from your rearing. That's a really great thing! That is what we strive for as parents. But it doesn't always happen that way. Sometimes the opinions of others were strong and miscommunicated. The original intention may have been positive, but as the message flowed downstream into your little mind, it was received as something entirely different. Often with the filter of, *I must not be good enough.*

I know for sure that I want to be my own woman, expressing myself from my personal beliefs and values. Not a parrot repeating what I've been told, or a puppet dancing a jig from another person's ideals. I believe that is how I have become a whole woman; by sorting through the opinions of others, the labels put on me as a child, and deciding for myself who I am. Wouldn't you like your beliefs to be your own, and not adopted from someone else? This health journey can be an empowering and life changing experience that gives you the ability to design your own life.

In his parable book, *The Ant and the Elephant,* respected author and Olympian Vince Poscente explains the relationship between the conscious and the subconscious mind, in my opinion, more simply and beautifully than anyone. He tells the story of Adir and Elgo both searching for meaning in their lives, and how they found hope and success in finding each other. The ant represents the conscious mind, and the elephant, the mighty and powerful subconscious. The little ant spends his whole life on a relentless journey to find the promised land, when he shockingly discovers his life's pursuit has been spent on the back of the elephant. It's a good read, and I highly recommend spending a quick two hours with it. It gives a metaphoric understanding of how the conscious and subconscious minds work together. You often spend so much time thinking it's your willpower that needs to change, while all along a much greater power is keeping you from achieving your goal.

Here's another way of thinking of it. Your mind is similar to operating a computer. The conscious mind is much like you sitting at your desk, manipulating the software and information in your computer. You decipher facts, add and delete, think in black and white, and make decisions based on the stored information. While your subconscious is like the hard drive. It does not analyze the information; it simply stores the content and makes it accessible when you need it. Imagine the hard drive content is all of your life experiences. Perhaps you experienced a controlling mother, or an abusive parent or family member—sexual, physical, emotional or otherwise. Maybe you had lack of a parent altogether, and experienced the hardships of that reality. From the lows of childhood adversity, to the highs of achievement throughout your rearing, both good and bad, all of it made an impression, and it is the stored data in your hard drive. The information and experiences that are stored in the subconscious mind, or your hard drive, have formed the foundation of your belief systems. These belief systems either propel you forward, or they hold you back.

When I was growing up I often heard the statement, "There are children starving in China. Eat everything on your plate. You cannot get up from the table until your plate is clean." Those words became engrained in my mind, and formed a powerful habit for me, finishing everything on my plate, always. As an adult this habit greatly contributed to overeating, which lead to weight gain. It's been a habit that is hard to shake loose simply because those words are an impression infused upon the walls of my mind. Can you relate?

Think about how powerful this concept is to your weight loss. My belief that I needed to eat everything on my plate was a message in my subconscious. It was my stored data. In my adult life, I knew that eating smaller meals, or stopping when I was full was the correct way to eat healthy. Yet, I found it very difficult to do, because my computer had old programming. For years, I had let my mom's beliefs become mine. Not intentionally, but subconsciously.

JANIE'S STORY

A client, we'll call her Janie for confidentiality sake, once said to me, "I can't get healthy. Everything I have tried just does not work. When I do lose weight, I gain it back. I guess I am destined to be fat just like my mom, my aunts, and my sisters. It's just our body type." Her words came from what she believed to be her truth, and her truth became her inability to getting healthy no matter what she tried. It's as if she sat down at her desk, and typed into her computer on Sunday.

This Week's To-Do List:

1. Start healthy eating plan on Monday
2. Exercise daily
3. Eat more vegetables

But, when she starts her good intentions on Monday, all of the stored content in her hard drive, her limiting belief systems and past failures, now come into play mode and sabotage her eating plan soon thereafter. The willpower to say no to sabotaging foods is just not enough. Janie feels discouraged when she blows it, and she believes she just can't do it, giving even more truth to her already limited belief about herself. But it's not Janie's fault, after all, she is merely working off of the information that is accessible to her. She is deriving from her existing hard drive. What is the definition of insanity? Doing the same thing over and over and expecting a different result. She cannot expect to change her outcome, unless she switches out the stored content on her hard drive. Janie needs new programming.

MOM'S STORY

When I was growing up, Mom and I had a tumultuous relationship. I now believe that it was a result of my parents divorcing at an early age. Mom was very angry and hurt by the divorce, and her emotions spilled over to my four-year-old receptive mind. Therefore, I became angry too. My resentful emotions were never directed towards Dad, but always like a boomerang of fury back at Mom. I did not feel like I had an outlet to express that rage, so Mom often received the brunt of it. In addition, Mom found it difficult to say, "I love you." Not just to me, but in general, and to all four of us kids. One can only guess that her inability to express her love verbally was derived from the way she was raised and her own hurts and pains. But nevertheless, I was a kid, and like all kids, I needed to be loved.

Although she did not say the words, "I love you," Mom did however express her love for us through baking. Just about every day, I would come home from school and be greeted by the smell of fresh baked chocolate brownies, chocolate chip cookies, lemon bars, or angel food cakes. It was like walking into a giant hug. It was her way of saying I love you. Ahhh ... the warmth of yummy treats for my tummy. Food instantly stimulates the senses. My receptors were open and storing the data. It wasn't long before I registered that food meant love. It was the easiest, fastest, most convenient way to self-soothe.

Kids need love, and I (snickering) loved myself often with food. My sister and I were eager to take on this baking love as well. We often pulled out all the ingredients for made-from-scratch chocolate chip cookies. But our cookie dough almost never made it to the oven. We'd eat the batter from the metal bowl by finger lick and spoonful until it was gone. We'd feel sick having ingested the unbaked cookies, but we'd do it again, time after time. I obviously didn't consciously realize these behaviors were being formed, otherwise I wouldn't have participated in a process that would cause so many years of grief. But this is the point. Our subconscious is powerful.

Thinking back over those younger years, I have realized my world was forming around me, and I was being molded by the unconscious data being collected. My belief systems were being shaped by how I perceived my family to feel about me. My friends, my circumstances, and my decisions were based on how I believed I fit into my world. There is a lot of room for error in that process. Many truths were not true at all, yet I perceived them to be my reality.

For me, food was not just for the basic need of keeping my body alive. It meant much more than that; it was a lifeline. It became part of me, and how I dealt with situations. As the years went by, I continued to use food for emotional stability. It wouldn't be until I was thirty years old that I made the connection. I don't have to use food for love, I can just love myself. Finally, as an adult woman, Ding, Ding, Ding! Bells are ringing, trumpets are blaring, light bulbs are blinking. Holy Cow, it was as if a veil had been lifted, and I could now see the light!

I learned this subconscious association from Mom. When she was dying, about three weeks from that final day, I went to visit her in the hospital. She had not eaten her lunch. On the tray sat her meat and veggies, along with a small salad. The one thing she did eat was her dessert. She always ate dessert. Throughout our adult lives, my sister and I would joke about Mom and her cinnamon rolls. Mom would go on one diet after another, refraining from her sweets for a period of time, but she couldn't hold out long. I'd say, "If we could just get her to stop eating cinnamon rolls, she might actually achieve something."

On that day, visiting her in the hospital, I finally learned what kept her relentlessly tied to her love of sweets. It wasn't just because sweets taste so darn good. I said, "Mom, why didn't you eat your lunch? You only ate the apple pie?" She answered in a blunt, sarcastic voice, "De'Anna, when you haven't had sex in 27 years, apple pie tastes really good."

My mouth dropped open. I couldn't believe it! Mom had never even uttered a word about sex my entire life. Mom never shared her emotions. Mom was so busy being critical of others that she made it incredibly hard for people to love her.

She just dropped the bomb. She finally revealed her subconscious association with sweets.

Sweets = Love and Intimacy.

Now we know food can't possibly provide real love and intimacy, but when you're in a highly emotional state and you decide to eat to numb those feelings, your subconscious mind begins to associate food with self-care. In that moment, and every moment that she chose to eat sweets, she was unconsciously thinking she was meeting her own needs. When she goes on a healthy eating plan and restricts her favorite sweets, it's as if she is NOT taking care of herself. Therefore, every attempt at getting healthy will fail.

HERE IS WHERE THE REAL GROWTH-WORK BEGINS

I encourage you to take a moment to examine your possible subconscious associations with food, and the old programming that might be playing in your head? Your story may be very different from mine or Mom's, but it's a sure bet that your current behaviors have roots that are long and embedded.

At the end of this, and throughout every chapter you have already discovered, there is an opportunity to engage in the process of rewriting your hard drive with the F.I.T. Session Exercises. I believe it is absolutely imperative that you make important mental shifts to your subconscious, in order to yield more positive results than you've been getting. We must recondition the mind to perceive a new you. Neuroscience tells us that our neuropathways are 100% capable to grow new neurons throughout life.

Think about how your history has developed your beliefs about yourself. How have life's influences over the years contributed to your body image, self-esteem, and eating habits? What were your parents' opinions, habits and beliefs?

F.I.T. EXERCISE

Before journaling this prompt, be sure to take a few deep inhales and exhales, allow the question to ruminate in your mind, close your eyes and let the answer bubble to the surface. Then open your eyes and write.

In regards to your weight and health, what are your initial thoughts about how you may have been programmed from your life's experiences?

_____

_____

_____

_____

_____

_____

You are holding the key in what's been keeping you from being successful permanently. It's not just about exercising your ass off like the biggest losers, or depriving yourself of your favorite foods for weeks on end. It's more than that. Anyone who has ever successfully changed their food intake, and actually kept extra weight off for good, has succeeded in changing their behaviors and self-identity. It was not the diet that helped them achieve their goal, it was the fact that they changed their belief systems as they also made better food choices, and created a schedule of regular exercise. They changed their old habits and formed a healthy new lifestyle.

Are you ready to face your inner belief systems, and shift them towards your highest good? If you said, "Yes!" ... let's get started. You must decide right now what your standards are for yourself. It is imperative that you begin to raise your bar. You must make YOU a priority in your life, and begin to feel worthy of the time you spend with yourself. You must also start caring about what and how much you eat, not because you're on a diet, but because YOU MATTER, and your health matters.

Science proves that to have lasting results at anything, a shift in consciousness must occur. In other words, it is vital that you revisit the issue from a different state of consciousness than the one that created it. So if you've had body weight struggles, and I imagine that is why you're reading this book, then you must do things differently than you've always done, in order to have new desired results. You must recreate your habits, and begin to live your life as who you want to be, rather than who you've been. Read that last line again, it is vital to your success. You must load new software in your hard drive.

I'm going to be super, straight-up honest with you. I have good news, and I have bad news.

The good news is, you're not the same person today that created the original bad habits that you've been working against. Remember at the beginning of this chapter, I stated, it's not really even your fault that you may be out of shape. You've just been working with the same old programming, the old hard data facts that predict the same results over and over.

Your subconscious mind has done its job well. It has carried out its duty to override any fleeting act of, *I'm going to be good with what I eat this week.* Your subconscious hard drive knows better, and is ready to kick in with its powerful old programming. Your subconscious mind is running off of the negative belief systems that are installed; the belief systems that your life experiences have created for you. The life experiences have been derived, not just from childhood, but all the other impressionable moments; divorce, death, trauma, stressful work-life, relationships that didn't work out, embarrassment, lack of worthiness and more. And that is the good news! You might be saying, "What? I don't follow, that's the good news?" Stay with me, you'll soon GET IT, I promise ...

Let's get on to the bad news. The bad news is, this is not going to happen overnight. I'm not going to tell you that you can lose 40 pounds in 4 weeks and keep it off. That's ridiculous! I refuse to be dishonest with you, and stoop to the level of the liars in the diet business. The social media memes, before and after photos and commercials, are full of empty promises that will only keep you spending your money on supplements and sabotaging your long-term success.

This is going to require your attention, and it's going to be totally worth it. Why? Because you're worth it. It may be one of the most challenging things you have experienced in your life. Not because it's hard, but because its been so easy to avoid. Be prepared, this process may send you on a journey exploring emotions, finding yourself one day in a pity of tears, and another at the breakthrough of victory. But that's because I am asking you to start feeling with your soul, rather than your stomach. It's high time you acknowledge yourself as worthy of having the healthy body you want. There may be moments through this process that you feel like you are hanging out of an airplane without a chute. And that will be great, because it means that you are being pushed from your comfort zone of doing what you've always done. In those moments, you are rewriting your hard drive. It will be worth your courage! So you see, it really is all GOOD NEWS!

Perhaps you are a person who doesn't even know where to begin with truly getting healthy. You've tried to be consistent but you're still back at square one. It's discouraging, you're confused and you're tired. Maybe some days you have an inkling of motivation, but it just feels too hard, and too time-consuming to devote your life to getting healthier.. You may even be a woman that's never even tried to diet, because you've resolved that you are simply built a certain way. Well I am here to declare, the body you want is developed from the inside out.

The reason it has felt like such a battle is because it is. You're up against that powerful machine we've been chatting about—your subconscious mind. If you don't have it working for you, then it will surely take control, and work against you. It's now up to you to delete the old bad habits, emotions and behaviors that do not serve you. You must input new information and resources, and deposit so much good stuff into your mind, that you begin taking action in new ways, and replacing the old thinking with a new powerful YOU.

Decide now that you are devoting your mind, body and soul to this process. It does not mean that getting healthy will have to take 100% of your time. However, it does mean that you must devote yourself in a new way. You've got to commit on a deeper level. This process is not about pussy-footing around (Ha! My mom use to say that) with eating healthier and dabbling in more exercise, and saying you're on a diet. BULLS*%T! This is like boot camp for your inner behaviors. You've got to step it up, and believe in YOU. Trust yourself through this process, and let's get to the ROOT so that you never have to diet again.

Are ya with me, girl? Good, let's do it together. I've got your back. I've done this myself, and write from my own experience. Even if you don't believe me yet, I know as your coach that YOU GOT THIS!

F.I.T. STRATEGY EXERCISE

Understanding You

This exercise will help you to recall your stored data. It is important that you bring the information that is filed through visualizations, feeling, and memory to the screen of your mind. Close your eyes, and ask your inner mind to access the associations you have regarding your history with food and body image. It is important that you put pen to paper, and let your hand express words through the thoughts that instantly come to your mind. This is not a time to analyze. That is the work of the conscious mind. This is an opportunity to express creatively from your subconscious aka "feeling" mind.

Close your eyes. Inhale and exhale five breaths.

What have I made food mean that it doesn't?

_____

_____

_____

_____

_____

_____

_____

_____

_____

_____

What are a few ways I can get my emotional needs met that are actually beneficial?

_____

_____

_____

_____

_____

_____

_____

_____

Ways I can feel fulfilled in my heart versus my stomach?

_____

_____

_____

_____

_____

_____

_____

Chapter 5 offers up important mindset techniques to your continued journey. You'll learn why you have been stuck in diet cycles, and how to adopt the mindset and behaviors that will align you with living as a F.I.T. Woman.

PART 2

COURAGE TO LOOK WITHIN

Chapter 5

It's a Mindset Thing

I think the key is for women not to set any limits.
~ Martina Navratilova

Mindset means that you have a particular way of viewing things in your life. It is grounded by your personal perspective. And that perspective has been shaped by the media, experiential fact, and from the influential people you've come in contact with throughout your lifetime. Having a positive mindset is absolutely a key component to sustaining a healthy life. But, positive mindset is only maintainable if you allow yourself breakthroughs. I am hopeful you've already experienced at least one breakthrough by interacting with this book thus far. Ready for your next one?

Through my own health journey, and the experience in working with the Mind Body F.I.T. women, I discovered a distinct difference between eating to lose weight and eating to be healthy. The mindset between the two perspectives are very different and also yield extremely opposite results.

First, let's turn our attention to the diet mindset. Let's be honest. Most weight loss programs call themselves a lifestyle, but they are truly a diet in disguise. But for those programs that really are great and focus on sustainability, it could be you showing up with a dieting mentality. We need to shift that line of thinking because it will keep you like a mouse on a wheel.

Let's address the diet mindset, or what I like to call the Fat Mindset, and explore its attributes. I believe diet and fat are one in the same. If you are always thinking you need to go on a diet, or you're trying to be good on your diet, then you must think, *I have weight to lose.* This type of thinking develops a mindset that is filled with harmful deceptions. It's not a nurturing place to be and definitely not a confidence-forming behavior.

When you go on a diet, it is as if you are planning for a beginning and an end. So if you start your diet on Monday, when does it end? Does it end when you blow it, and you need to get back on your diet? How many times have you said, "I'll start on Monday." There is a definitive timeline to the diet mindset. It is a temporary means to a goal that has many downfalls. This is how we become trapped in yo-yo dieting.

How often have you set a goal for yourself to lose X amount of body in X amount of weeks? With the best of intentions, you buy all the good food at the grocery store. You start working out extra hard, and you even do it religiously. After all, you have a goal to achieve, right? You may have set that goal because your high school reunion is coming up, and you really want to impress the people you haven't seen for years. Maybe you're getting married, and you have a certain idea in your mind about how you want to look on your wedding day. You are on a mission to achieve weight loss in a measurable amount of time, so you do everything in your power to make that goal a reality. You have dangled the carrot (pun intended), and you are focused.

While dieting, think about all the extra time you have put into exercising. You may have made it such a priority that you turned down outings and fun things with friends or family. You say, "Oh no, I can't, I've got to work out today." A couple months later you miraculously reach your goal body and feel great about yourself. You temporarily worked hard, focused on eating better, warded off the cravings ... oh, but wait, what happens after that time period?

Let's think about this for a moment. Never once did you consider what will happen after you say, "I do." You just figure that everything will be great because you hit your goal weight, and it will all just take care of itself. Never once did you think beyond the wedding day, and strategize your body maintenance for the future. You simply put your focus on a segment of time. Aha! A trap! Sorry to have to say it like this, but you are hallucinating! There's more ...

Soon you decide that you're feeling so good about yourself and you look so great, that you can have a Caramel Macchiato again. You can reward yourself! Yippeee! That's how it starts. But then, sneaking back into your life is the dreaded recourse. A stressful incident happens as life is sure to serve it up when you least expect it, and your stored old data of turning to food begins to creep back into your days. First just a little and then a lot. As time goes by you slowly go back to your old habits and end up gaining the weight back. You're left disgusted, disappointed and wishing for your skinny jeans to fit you again. Whew ... it's all so exhausting, isn't it?

If you have not engaged in yo-yo dieting, perhaps you have experienced a Fat Mindset in other ways. Many of my clients have succumbed to their subconscious messages and formed mindsets that they are just going to be overweight—because it's how they are made. Because of the messages they have received by life; feeling out of place because of their body, being ridiculed and categorized or the media telling us that we gain five pounds a year as we age. You have made up your mind that this is "who you are."

Our minds are so powerful that we can literally create beliefs and mindsets about ourselves, and it becomes how we live our lives. Everything we do is rooted from that point of view. When you are dieting, you have a powerless mindset. There are many restrictions you put on yourself while on a diet, wouldn't you agree? You can't have this, and you can't have that. You are weak to temptations because you've told yourself, "No." You have to measure your food, you have to count calories, and you are instilled with the feeling of deprivation. All of which are for the sole purpose of losing weight in a relatively short amount of time. The choices are taken from you, and the feeling of "I have to" sets in.

I have to go exercise.

I can't have mayo on my sandwich.

Hold the bun; I can't have that. Too many carbs.

No thank you: I can't have it; I'm on a diet.

You are helpless against a much stronger force. You can only stick with it for a short period of time. You feelin' me girl? Are we on the same wavelength? Think about how much time we spend working out for a particular goal. If all of that working out is not realistic to a lifestyle for you, then it is just not something you can keep up. You will get burned out, and you will quit.

For example: a client of mine shared with me that when she was on a program—let's call it Weight Lookers—she adhered to the eating plan very closely and focused on clocking X amount of steps on her pedometer each day. She became so obsessed with increasing those registered numbers that practically all she was doing was walking, walking and walking just to beat her own daily records. While beating records is great, and all in due time, what happened to my client is, she became overwhelmed by the demand of her unrealistic expectations. She couldn't keep up with the high standards she set for herself. Eventually she stopped walking altogether, and gained back all of the weight she lost. Now she's back at square one and joining my program.

Here's the irony: her first inkling once she joined the MBFC program was to dust off her pedometer and start the whole madness over again. This is a diet cycle, a Fat Mindset. Had she focused on a reasonable amount of exercise each day, she'd still be doing it, and she would have maintained her body easily breaking the vicious cycle of the past.

Often I have had women say to me, "I'll work out with you once I lose some weight." That is ridiculously backwards, don't ya think? But a Fat Mindset thinks of the "fit people" as a different breed; they can't help but think that way because they have conditioned themselves to do so. Have you had a fit friend invite you to go walking or for a jog? And you make up an excuse, or flat out say, "No way," because you are either scared you'll keel over, or simply aren't interested at all in jogging because you think, *Big girls don't jog.* Countless times I have heard new Mind Body F.I.T. Club women express their feelings of intimidation of going to the gym. They feel like all eyes are on them "the fat girl on the treadmill."

While running a half marathon, I came upon a girl vomiting on the side of the road. When I asked if she was okay, she answered, "Yeah, it's just nerves." I asked her what her anxiety was about. She said, "I just want to finish." As I probed her and asked more questions, she divulged that she had all the negative messages of her life circling in her head. She thought about how many times she was ridiculed for being fat, and how the overall message from society is that *fat girls don't run.* She was on mile 5 out of 13, and she was running. Yet, her mental language was so strong that it made her physically sick, and she doubted her performance. On that day, she was choosing to listen to her old programming.

The negative language we allow ourselves to engage in is really all nonsense that we've made up in our minds. So how do you get out of this trap and start to shape your mind with purposeful intention? How do you get rid of old thinking and create new perspectives? I'm about to share it with you, and it will be easier than you might think.

To become a F.I.T. Woman, you have to think and act like one NOW! We as humans are prone to habitual behavior. We like it; we live by it through repetitive routines and schedules. Having a certain method of how we do things makes us feel safe and comfortable. Repetition in our lives is predictable and measurable. Without repetition we are living in the unknown, and that can be scary. As much as repetition dictates our old habits, repetition is also a key factor in creating new habits. When we do something new, we initially feel uncertain and question our ability. Yet the more we repeatedly practice, the better we get, and soon we feel comfortable with the new habit.

This is a method for developing a new mindset. Repeat a new behavior over and over until it becomes natural to you. It will become unconscious after a period of time, and then your efforts will be relieved to something that just feels normal for you to do. You won't have to consciously focus on it anymore; it becomes just how you do things. This practice only works if the behavior you are working to build is sustainable. In other words, if you cannot maintain the level of time you devote to the new habit, then it is not a habit that will stay with you.

The idea I really want you to take to the bank is this: utilize the methodology that repeated daily, healthful acts will cause a shift in mindset, and result in a BODY YOU LOVE. And by participating in this repeated behavior, you will strategically align yourself with attracting the support and guidance you need to make the mindshift concrete. As you seek change, new insight will come to you in the form of fitness enthusiasts and educators; people who have been successful at maintaining health, and supportive programs; all because it is your focused interest, and your awareness is open to learning more. Dieters can easily transition into the nutritionally conscious, and non-movers can transform into fitness enthusiasts.

The F.I.T. Mindset Creates a Feeling of Power

The F.I.T. Mindset gives you back your personal power. It offers up a boundless amount of choices. You can make the decision to shift your thinking from I can't, and instead, choose to be the I can miracle.

I am choosing to eat healthier.

I am choosing to consume foods that give me more energy.

I am choosing to exercise because I know I'll feel good afterward.

I am choosing to let go of old cravings because I know they did not serve my highest good.

I am choosing to understand my emotions better, and make conscious decisions.

I am living as the woman I want to be.

I am learning to meet my emotional needs in new and effective ways.

I am in the process of returning to my natural and ideal weight.

In the F.I.T. Mindset you are choosing to take a POWERFUL position in your body's health. You hold all the cards. You become proactive, mindful, and strategic. This is the mindset of the F.I.T. Woman! She commands her mind.

PAM'S STORY

I'd like to share with you a story about a girl named Pam. (In respect of her privacy, I have changed her given name to a different three letter name.) She became part of The Mind Body F.I.T. Club community because she had a burning desire to get healthy and in shape. Pam grew up challenged with body issues; she was raised in an obese family and suffered from many physical ailments. She had a plethora of circumstances against her in her battle to get her body under control. Over a period of time between the ages of 19-21 she had five knee surgeries. Her friends and family became accustomed to seeing her on crutches, and she became the girl with the knee injury. Fast forward a decade or so. When she entered the Mind Body F.I.T. Club, she had a total of eight knee surgeries. She began at Day 1 with hope in her heart that this would be the program that would help her change her life and finally get to a healthy weight she could sustain.

Pam excitedly moved through the self-development materials by answering and journaling the given daily questions. She also repetitively listened to the F.I.T. Session audios and became a regular on our coaching calls. Through creating a new awareness, Pam began to realize that she had built a mindset around her knee problems. She discovered that all of these years she had used her ailing knees as her excuse to not getting healthy. She would often find herself turning down exercise by saying, "No I can't. I have bad knees." One day it dawned on Pam that she had been defining herself through her knee problems. Her bad knees became who she was. Everything in her life revolved around her injuries, her surgeries and what she couldn't do.

Pam had not made the connection until it was reflected back to her through our program materials. Once she cleared the fog and grew her AWARENESS, Pam was able to bring the unconscious behaviors out into the open. It was like a whole new world opened up in her mind. She was able to shift an old mindset into a brand new F.I.T. Mindset that she had never known before. An OMG moment!

Pam had lived her entire life within walking distance to her local YMCA. Never once over the years had she set foot in that gym or even thought of it as a place for her to go. Now that she is enlightened with new self-understanding, she not only joined the Y, but you can find her there more than half the week. Pam has lost over forty pounds and now considers herself a fitness enthusiast. She is an inspiration to everyone who knows her. She regularly enjoys spinning, swimming and even belly dancing classes. Perhaps you want to know, does Pam still have knee issues? Yes she does, but she figures they hurt before anyway, even when she did nothing. She says, "I might as well be in shape and feel good about myself. And if my knees hurt, well, at least they hurt on a thinner, fit body." Pam continues to impress us all with her amazing shift in mindset.

The F.I.T. Mindset Woman looks for ways to be active in both her free time and her scheduled time. Moving her body becomes an activity she loves. If you're a woman who dreads exercise, I am asking you to open your mind to the possibilities rather than focus on your self-induced limitations. Put one foot in front of the other, and direct your attention to one a day at a time. See the possibilities for being active as opportunities!

Once exercise becomes a more habitual part of who you are, you'll find that meeting others who exercise is easy, that's when the real fun and adventure begins! The Mind Body F.I.T. Club ladies are exuberant about participating in organized events like 5K, 10K, half marathons and triathlons. When we participate in events together, we cheer, holler, and give out lots of "Atta Girls!" And by doing so, it becomes a memorable and very fun experience. Keep in mind, these are women just like you. They haven't always been athletes, but they are learning that they can be. When you socialize with others who are living a lifestyle of health, it is a great influence on you. We've already talked about how the influences you've had in the past are responsible for forming beliefs and behaviors you have now. Perhaps it's time for some new fit friends! These people come in various shapes and sizes, yet they have a commonality. Their unity is taking care of themselves through awareness of their nutrition, regular exercise, and taking personal responsibility for their health. Dieting is not how they live their life; it's truly about health.

Are you starting to get the mindshift I am presenting to you? Embracing a F.I.T. perspective now will give you new and desired results. The process is pain-free, all you have to do is let go of the old you. Sometimes we hold on to our old ways merely because it's what we know. But as Oprah says, "Now that you know, you can't say you don't know." Take the steps forward to welcome change. Taking better care of yourself doesn't have to be so darn hard. So why make it that way?

Choose to take on the F.I.T. Mindset now, and watch yourself morph into a new woman. Adopt the strategies written here, and repeat them on a daily basis. It's as simple as making choices for your health and well-being, and repeat, repeat, repeat.

THE F.I.T. WOMAN MINDSET

- Begin to enjoy exercise, and purposely engage in activity that is fun and sustainable over time.

- Hang out with people who take care of themselves. Watch them closely. If they can do it, so can YOU.

- Have the courage to examine the areas of your life that are not working for you. Identify unconscious habits and create awareness. Be honest with yourself.

- Divide your bad habits from your identity. You are not your bad habits. Your habits are what you do, not who you are. Who you are is your essence, your talents, and abilities. Start focusing on what you CAN do.

- Set attainable short-term goals that can later transition to *Lifestyle*. A F.I.T. Mindset looks beyond a regimented timeline.

At the end of the Mind Body Fit program, it states: "Welcome to the first day of the rest of your life." We can print such a claim because I know that if you plug-in, fully participate in the strategies given, and create new habits, you will discover your spirit and make the all important transition into a F.I.T. lifestyle. Welcome to the first day of the rest of your life.

F.I.T. STRATEGY EXERCISE

Inner F.I.T. Woman Visualization

To start living fit now, you must reprogram your subconscious thoughts to align with the F.I.T. Woman you want to become. Here you will use a creative process to help you unconsciously speak directly to your inner mind.

— Step 1 —

With paper and pencil, rally up your inner artist and draw how you believe you look now. That's right, include the bumps, and love handles. Don't worry about being a da Vinci. Draw yourself from your perspective to the best of your ability.

— Step 2 —

Next, draw the woman you want to be on the inside of your current parameters. Draw her with the lean curves and strong body that you want. Have fun with your drawing by tapping into your playful inner child. This is not a time to pass judgment; it is an opportunity to dream.

— Step 3 —

The space between. Take a moment to observe the space between who you are now, and the **F.I.T. Woman** you want to become. The space between is an opportunity to learn, grow and develop. Along the left side of your Inner F.I.T. Woman drawing, describe what the space between represents.

What poor habits created the space between?

_____

_____

_____

_____

What emotions must be released to unveil the **F.I.T. Woman** inside of you?

_____

_____

_____

_____

_____

List any feelings of unworthiness, past hurts, pains or experiences that have been weighing you down.

_____

_____

_____

_____

_____

— Step 4 —

The F.I.T. Woman profile. On the right side of your drawing, create a profile of the success factors of the F.I.T. Woman. Think as if you are that beautiful F.I.T. Woman and project the answers from 'her' point of view.

What does your **F.I.T. Woman** eat for energy?

_____

_____

_____

_____

What is her schedule like? Does she create time to exercise and plan her meals?

_____

_____

_____

_____

How does she relax?

_____

_____

_____

_____

How does she handle stress?

_____

_____

_____

_____

_____

How do others respond to her?

_____

_____

_____

_____

What activities does she do for fun?

_____

_____

_____

_____

How does she feel about herself?

_____

_____

_____

_____

_____

— Step 5 —

Take a good look at the F.I.T. Woman attributes and decide to apply them to your life now. Have faith and trust in yourself. Rely on your Inner F.I.T. Woman as guidance in helping you to make better decisions.

In a moment of food-distraction, before you choose to eat the creamy pasta, ask yourself, *What choice would my Inner F.I.T. Woman make? The pasta or the healthy salad with lean protein?*

In a moment of struggle, before you dig into the ice cream to soothe stress, ask yourself, *How would she choose to react? Would she eat to self-soothe, or would she get some exercise to de-stress?*

Adopt the behaviors of your Inner F.I.T. Woman now. Don't wait. This process is like a map guiding you to your desire. It engages your immediate thinking and subconscious programming. Even better, it helps you to shift your internal paradigms; believing that you can achieve your ultimate goal. Now in no way does this exercise suggest that if you are thinner or weigh less you are more worthy. It is simply a way of showing you (versus telling you) that your self-identity and the habits you attach to that make a difference in how you take care of yourself.

In the next chapter, you'll read the story of a girl who displays a revealing amount of courage on her persistent path to overcoming her lifelong body issues. I ask you to associate your own reasons and beliefs that reveal your untold story. Continue with courage.

Chapter 6

Belief Breakthroughs

*Move to the rhythm of your soul and
you'll never miss a beat.*

~ Vicki Virk

Worthiness. Ah yes, we are going to go there. Now this emotion runs deep, doesn't it? Ask yourself, do I truly feel worthy of having the body I say I want? On the surface you might sarcastically answer, "Yeah, De'Anna, otherwise I wouldn't be reading your book." But when it comes down to it, do you really feel like you can successfully maintain a healthy body and BE that woman?

Although you say you want to get healthy now, you may have doubt that creeps in as you continue your journey. Self-limiting beliefs may surface, and be disguised as obstacles in your path. Those obstacles can feel legitimate. They can feel as real as the surface you are sitting on. But they're not real. They are made up of all that we have talked about; the representations of the past mental pictures, people and experiences that your mind has packaged, and molded into your personal belief systems.

You can break through! The phrase-people don't change. It's not true. People do change. I see it happen for my clients consistently. The change happens through our deeper Hypnotherapy work as well as the risks they begin taking because of the self-growth they experience. It is awe-inspiring. Courage and consciousness make miracles happen.

GENELLE'S STORY

I'd like to share with you a story of a woman whom I admire greatly. Her name is Genelle. She is a feisty woman in her mid-forties that became my client by chance. Well, let me rephrase that. I don't believe in accidental, chance meetings, but I do believe in the twist *of fate* kind. So, we'll safely say that she and I met because it was in our stars.

Before meeting Genelle in person, she spent many sequential days listening to my voice. Let me explain. My husband, Troy, had met her while out running an errand to her boat shop. Genelle was there, and he overheard her talking to a client about quitting smoking. He told Genelle that he had something that could help her quit. He quickly ran out to his truck, grabbed one of my *Hypnosis SmokeFree* audios, brought it into her and said, "Here, just listen to it." Although she admits she had been skeptical about it working, she did faithfully listen to it, and she did successfully quit smoking within a month. We had never met, yet the sound of my voice, and the positive, hypnotic words that I said on the program were distinctive in her mind.

About a year later, we were soaking in the beautiful mountain sun one summer afternoon during a family day of boating. We were floating in North Bay with friends, when my husband spotted Genelle on her boat across the sparkling water. He dove in, and swam over 200 feet to her boat to say hello. He hung out with her and friends for a bit, and enjoyed a cold brew. In his persuasive manner, my husband convinced Genelle to come over and meet me in person. She was hesitant. She was thinking perhaps I could hypnotize her without her knowing, and maybe I would play weird tricks with her mind. As untrue as that is (being a Hypnotist, I get that a lot), she was a bit nervous. The *SmokeFree* audio had worked well for her, and she felt that she had become conditioned to my voice. So the thought of meeting me in person freaked her out a little. Reluctantly she kicked her way across the cool summer water and introduced herself. She was a beautiful woman with long blondish hair and eyes the color of the sea. We made our formal introductions and segued into chatting casually. When I heard about her reservations with meeting me, it gave me a good laugh. Often I find, people have misunderstood perceptions of hypnosis. I reassured her that I always have the best intentions in mind, and I would not hypnotize her knowingly or unknowingly without her participation.

After that chance meeting, a few months later, Genelle became my client once again, but this time for weight loss. I was excited. After all, I knew she had experienced great results with quitting smoking. Getting her into my program was thrilling. I love to see the products I create work effectively for people, and I was happy to have her in the Mind Body F.I.T. Program. I was very hopeful she would have a positive outcome.

As I got to know Genelle, I was quick to learn she was a Type A personality to the max. She had interesting dynamics; although she was a real goal achiever, she also had a lifelong struggle with her body. I remember thinking curiously, here we have a woman who is very successful in her career, runs a company, is well organized, and has the mindset that she can successfully tackle any project that is dropped on her desk. But yet, she has not learned to apply these skills to weight management. I knew she had something subconscious going on hindering her and that made me even more eager to help.

In my experience, every woman who signs up for the Mind Body F.I.T. Programs is excited and enthusiastic about creating more energy, increasing confidence and dropping unnecessary pounds. Genelle was no different. I shared with her as I do all women joining, "This is not a diet, it is a process of learning about yourself, and understanding the roots of your behaviors so you can move forward more successfully." The tools and strategies I supply my ladies with help them to learn to focus on themselves, on the inside, and the weight loss becomes a secondary natural result of this powerful process. Once Genelle understood this formula could be the answer to figuring out her challenges, she fully engaged and plugged herself into the program. Of course she would, it's her personality to do so. She was a model student, open to personal development and willing to make strategic changes. Little did I know, in an effort to help her change her life, Genelle would change my life as well.

I was floored by the courage Genelle displayed to unravel her intricately woven belief systems that often limited her. That's certainly not an easy thing to do. Her spirited nature reminded me of my own fight to find myself, and I was often in awe of her perseverance. On more than one occasion we discussed the observed comparison; losing weight the right way is like peeling back the layers of an onion. There are many reasons why we choose to eat for the wrong reasons, operate from quick fixes, and withhold true success.

Genelle was a woman who displayed ultra-success in other areas of her life, but was debilitated when it came to weight control. Through coaching and guidance, Genelle took on an attitude of relentless pursuit in search of the answer to her most daunting question. *Why is it that I have a weight problem?* We had numerous conversations, group coaching calls, and emails about the fact that her issue, like many others, was not just about the food she put into her mouth. It was about *Why?* Why did she sabotage herself on the weekends by inhaling an entire plate of rice Crispy Squares? It was certainly not because she was hungry. Why did she feel the need to eat that cupcake, and one more after that? It was definitely not because it was mealtime.

Genelle worked hard at pulling off her invisible mask to understand her struggle. She spent time sifting through her associations with food on an emotional and mental level, while simultaneously stepping up to the many physical challenges that I proposed to her. In a relatively short amount of time, through physical and mental training, Genelle was able to complete our Loop the Lake Challenge (a 15 kilometer loop around Lake Arrowhead, CA). It took a commitment of regular walking for her to build up the stamina and endurance to complete the challenge. She did it, and was very proud of her accomplishment. That she committed to the next challenge: a half marathon. I offer these challenges in our programs for a very specific reason. There are incredible mental shifts that naturally occur while simultaneously becoming more fit.

The strategy for the half marathon Genelle participated in, the Carlsbad Marathon, was simple; just finish. There was no time limit involved. The only pressure that Genelle felt was what she put on herself; her own mental state was questioning her ability to complete the race. The anxiety was somewhat relieved knowing she could walk the whole thing, and still win a medal. Yet going into it she was still nervous.

She felt incredibly uplifted by the experience. The fact that there were women just like her participating, and the support of onlookers cheering words of encouragement, were moments of pure positive energy. Genelle completed the race on that day with our exuberant Carol, a fellow Mind Body F.I.T. member, as they skipped, jumped and cheered their way down the last fifty yards toward the finish line. A marathon representative placed Genelle's well-earned medal over her head, and it was tangible proof that she did something great with her body that day. Not only was it a symbol of her hard-earned training, completing her walking week by week, but more importantly, her medal was a gift for her soul, a reminder of how important she is to herself. She could have made other things priority in her life. But she didn't. She committed to the training, followed through to her goal, and it was worth it. She was able to do that while simultaneously upholding her other work and life obligations. As a result of her new confidence, her career leadership skills blossomed as well.

Now during her experience that day at the Carlsbad Marathon, Genelle had glanced at a bystander's sign that read, "Remember, you're doing it for the Triple Crown!" That visual stuck in her head, so a few days after the race, she went online to investigate. She researched the details and learned that those who complete three specific half marathons within a calendar year would be eligible for a fourth special status medal—The Triple Crown. Genelle had caught the marathon medal bug with that very first one, and knew she wanted more medals, and more challenging experiences. She was determined to win her battle with weight and use the half marathons as a means to abolish any self-limiting behaviors. Without any hesitation, she signed up for the next race that would qualify her for the Triple Crown— the La Jolla Half Marathon. What she did not know is the La Jolla Half Marathon is an infamous race, known for its hilly, challenging course. Amongst the many hills is the notorious Torrey Pines hill that goes straight up from sea level to a three hundred foot plus ocean bluff. To top it off, not only was this course very intimidating, it also had a time limit.

Unknowingly, Genelle had signed up for a life-challenging experience. Once again, Genelle trained hard. She worked with a personal trainer, and physically and mentally pushed herself through barriers knowing the pressure was on to improve. All the while, she knew she must finish the next race 30 minutes faster than the last one in order to receive a medal. That meant she had to learn to move her body at a faster pace; instead of walking a 16-minute mile, she had to jog a 13-minute mile. This was no small feat. Genelle was 220 pounds, and had signed on to carry herself up and down 13 plus hilly miles. A very difficult task!

Genelle's sister, Jaylene, and I excitedly agreed to accompany her to the La Jolla Half Marathon. I would be along her side as her personal mental coach, and Jaylene would be her faithful fan club cheering her on, taking pictures to document her accomplishment. The night before the race, she lay staring at the clock, unable to sleep. The anxiety was so strong, her thoughts filled with, *What if I don't make it in time?* Her worst nightmare was being swept by the bus. Being swept is when you are picked up along the course for not finishing within the allotted time. As soon as she heard me stirring in the wee morning hour, she came running into my room, and jumped onto my bed. Nerves had kept her awake the whole night, and she was ready to go get this race started and over with.

When we arrived at 6 a.m. to the crowded parking lot, runners were gathering their water bottles and gear from their cars, and heading to the start line. The three of us sat in the car for a few moments. Genelle's eyes welled with tears as she started to cry. She was feeling overwhelmed by fear as she looked around. She saw, from her point of view, all of these fit-looking people getting out of their cars. They were warming up and preparing for the race by jogging through the parking lot. She felt very out of place, and highly intimidated as if she did not have a right to be there. Genelle was downright scared.

We made our way from the parking lot to the start line amongst the 6,000 plus runners. As we awaited the gun shot, I turned to Genelle, and wrapped my arms around her. I asked her to close her eyes, and I whispered, "You earned your right to be here. You are a fighter, a warrior, and I believe in you. It does not matter whether you get a medal today, what matters most is that you have chosen to be in the race. You have proven to yourself that you are in this to win this for you." Our meditational pep talk ended with tears and a group hug with Jaylene.

The gunshot went off, and we slowly jogged away from Jaylene and the start line. At just mile one Genelle was breathing hard and turning shades of red. Although I knew she had trained for this day, her physical responses made me wonder if perhaps she had taken on more than she could truly handle. I knew it had to be her mental state, so I reassured her that her body was warming up, she would be feeling fine a few miles down the road and to just take it slow. She later divulged that she was feeling so much fear within that first mile of the race that she wanted to fake an injury by falling down and claiming she twisted her ankle or pretend she was having a seizure. We've since laughed out loud about that many times.

About four miles down the road, we spotted a woman about 15 yards ahead. This woman had an extremely voluptuous backside, and I mean she had booooooooty. And, by gosh, she was treading ahead at a slow but consistent pace. She did not have the body of a lean runner, nor did she closely resemble the vision of a 'marathoner.' Yet, there she was, alone, in the race and moving down the asphalt one step at a time. She was a badass. As I looked ahead at this woman, my eyes filled with tears, and my throat choked up as I thought to myself, *My Gosh, this woman has the heart of a winner, just like the Kenyan coming in first place at this race. She has every bit the mindset of a champion, giving it her all.*

I felt so impressed by her and emotionally moved by her courage.

In that same moment, I looked over and observed Genelle. Her face was flushed and she was carrying her body as if she was getting tired. We still had the big Torrey Pines hill ahead of us to defeat. She needed motivation to keep her legs moving and her mind on the finish line, so I pointed at the courageous woman in front of us and said, "Genelle, you do not let her out of your sight. If she can do this, so can you."

Through her doubtful thinking, Genelle immediately responded by saying, "You don't know De'Anna, maybe she runs all the time, maybe she's in better shape than me." Rolling my eyes, I said to Genelle with sarcasm, "Oh please, in no way is she in better shape than you. Just get your ass moving." Perhaps my words come across harsh on paper. You must know that Genelle and I have a funny, sarcastic connection. She got the message, and knew it was correct. She did have the strength, and so did the woman ahead of her. It comes down to having the mindset to recognize it and charge ahead. She did just that.

At about mile five we started up the bottom of the tall and threatening Torrey Pines Hill. I had a sneaky strategy up my sleeve to help Genelle with her climb. I knew she had created a huge obstacle in her mind about this hill; she was full-blown intimidated. Quite honestly, it is a really big hill, but Genelle had transformed Torrey Pines hill into Mt. Everest in her mind. Without Genelle seeing what I was up to, I pulled my phone out from under my shirt. I got it ready with the perfect song, hit play and placed the ear buds in her ears. Blasting in her head, forcing her to go internal, was that old Alicia Keys song "Superwoman." Alicia affirming to Genelle as if it were her own thoughts.

When I'm breaking down and I can't be found

As I start to get weak

'Cause no one knows me underneath these clothes

But I can fly, we can fly, oh

'Cause I am a Superwoman

Yes I am, Yes she is

Even when I'm a mess, I still put on a vest

With an S on my chest

Oh Yes, I'm a Superwoman

She started to almost hyperventilate as she became emotional listening to the words of that song. It was a moment amongst many moments that day that were special for Genelle. She identified with that song. It resonated with her because she was fighting the good fight to win her battle with herself, her own internal struggle to BE her full potential. My devious plan worked. She got herself up that dang mountain with what looked like, and I'm not kidding, the strength of a lion. Her face was determined and focused as if she was hunting her prey. She's like that in business, too! I was so proud of her. In true Genelle style, when she reached the top, she walked to the edge of the cliff and started beating her chest like Tarzan as she shouted out a big "AAAEEEEAAAAEEEAAAAA!!!" Hahaha, what a goofball this woman is, I love it.

Understanding Your Why

Genelle's intimidating hill was behind her, and we had five miles to the finish line. She and I were jog/walking along at a decent pace with the focus of just putting one foot in front of the other and getting the miles under our feet. Genelle had been working really hard to get healthy over the past year. She was exercising consistently, writing in her Mind Body F.I.T. Journal, listening to the F.I.T. Session audios, learning about nutrition ... doing everything she could to create success.

Frustratingly, she was still, on occasion, sabotaging her eating. She'd had an episode just a month or so back where she devoured a number of chocolate truffles, and then hid the wrappers in the couch so her then-husband wouldn't know. Now let me be clear. It's perfectly acceptable to eat chocolate. This story is not about not eating chocolate. It's about the obsessive emotional aspect of eating the chocolate. That is what we are focused on dissolving. While pacing beside her, the thought of her unconscious sabotages came to my mind. I wanted to know why. After all the work and effort she has put into transforming herself, why does she still impair her success?

Let's qualify sabotage. It's one thing to eat a truffle. After all, we are not promoting restriction or dieting, and chocolate should be a part of your lifestyle if that's your thing. We're talking a truffle binge. That's different. I knew we had built a real trust with each other, and it was not imposing to ask. I wanted to ask her this question while she had her defenses down. She was tired, and pushing hard to finish the race. I intuitively just knew this was the perfect time to ask her this very tough question. We were jogging along a tree line straightaway at mile 8 when I turned to Genelle and said, "Can I ask you a question? And please know that I ask with the utmost respect."

She kind of giggled, and hesitantly said, "Yeah." I said, "Why do you eat the chocolates?" Genelle answered, "I don't know."

Now of course, the chocolates, were just one example. What's important to remember, is the chocolates could be many different foods on various occasions. So the question was more of a metaphor than anything else, and she knew that. Unsatisfied with her answer, I asked again with a bit more strength in my voice, "Genelle, why do you eat the freakin' chocolates?" Once again she answered, "I don't know, D."

I said, "Yeah, you do know. Why do you sabotage yourself, why do you eat the chocolates?" And to my excitement, next she answered, "I don't know ... cause I'm not worthy." Ooohhh, now that's a telling answer. *Now we're getting somewhere,* I thought.

My personal experience as well as working with people, tells me that she doesn't just happen to feel less than worthy for no reason at all. There are roots to her self-limiting belief. My instinct told me that someone, at some point in her life, gave her that message—and I was determined to get to the bottom of it. Remember also, that an answer like that is in direct conflict with who she is at work and in life. This is a super successful woman and for her to feel unworthy deep down inside is most definitely an indicator of something old she's holding on to.

I said to Genelle, "Who told you that? Who told you that you're not worthy?" She reluctantly answers, "Eric." I'm thinking, *Who the heck is Eric?* I had gotten to know Genelle extremely well in our time working together, and I had never heard about some dude named Eric.

Genelle began to let out the pent-up feelings about her first marriage. Eric had abused her both mentally and physically. Over and over he would tell her she was worthless, fat and that no one would love her. He scared her. One time he even tied her up in a sheet and put her in the closet. After repeated abuse, Genelle began to believe his lies. Although she did save her own life and eventually empowered herself to leave him, Genelle internalized his dark messages and built an unconscious belief system to support them. Although he was physically gone, on the inside there was part of her that was left feeling unworthy.

I knew it was time for her to let all of that ugliness go. After all, that old Genelle was no longer aligning with the Genelle that was jogging next to me. She had grown; she was not the same person anymore. The woman I knew was strong and unstoppable and wouldn't let someone else's words hold her back. Finally, after all this time, I began to understand Genelle's body struggle. She had extra emotional baggage that needed to be left behind before she could move forward to the next level of her life. I felt clutched with emotion. I took a risk, and carefully voiced my opinion.

I said, "I don't see Eric here running this half marathon with you. He's not here because you left his sorry ass years ago. Because you are strong. You were too strong for Eric to hold you down then, and you're too strong to let him continue to do it now. You're a fighter, and it's time to let Eric go. He lied to you. He wanted to bring you down 'cause he felt like shit about himself, and he wanted you to feel that way too. Dammit Genelle, you are worthy. It's time to take back your power! You deserve it. You've earned your right to be here."

As we jogged down the race course, our eyes filled with tears. In that moment, our communication created a shift in consciousness for Genelle. The day of total renewal had arrived. Wanting to leave the past behind, she made a concrete decision to unconditionally love herself from that point forward. Through silent words, there was a feeling in the air that was unexplainable. A kind of soulful magic happened, as if heaviness was lifted from Genelle's spirit. She felt it, and I felt it too. It was a supernatural spiritual instance, a moment that we will both treasure forever.

Genelle began living her life from a new perspective from that day on. Had she not chosen to step out and take on the Triple Crown challenge, she may have not received this gift for her soul. Genelle later talked about the experience to friends and Mind Body F.I.T. members. She summed up that moment, and the overall day in these words, "The sky has turned a different shade of blue."

SO, WHO OR WHAT, IS YOUR 'ERIC'?

The true key to getting F.I.T. is having the courage to unlock the secrets you have hidden inside. The feelings of unworthiness, self-doubt, the ruminating questions of, "Do I deserve to have the body I want?" We all have people or experiences of our past that represent 'Eric.' As we've talked about in previous chapters, it could be childhood struggles, a relationship gone wrong, you name it. We all carry the weight of our lives. But you don't have to anymore.

In doing this amazing work that I feel absolutely privileged to be a part of, I have found that some people overeat to protect themselves from the emotional pain they don't want to feel. Others sabotage themselves with food because inside they don't feel worthy of having the body they want. Some women just don't commit on a deeper level, and give up before they see results. They mask their negative behaviors with a variety of excuses as to why they can't get healthy. They convince themselves that their reasons are justifiable, all because it's scary to face the truth. And often the truth is, *I don't deserve it.*

I get it, there is a plethora of challenges that you face in your battle. But, I'm going to share with you the real deal. Are you ready? Time and time again, my work has proven that there is really only one simple concept that every woman, no matter what their story, must wrap their brain around in order to have lasting weight loss.

Focus on YOU first, the body second.

YOU must understand what makes you tick.

Why do I eat when I'm not hungry?

Why did I let myself go?

Why don't I make me important in my day?

Once you make amends with your why, then making exercise a part of your lifestyle and eating for health becomes easy and secondary. Taking ownership of your *why* will create a new level of acceptance, so you can take responsibility and move on.

Start making yourself a priority today. Take the time to think about your limiting beliefs. Have the courage to shift them by creating daily thinking habits that remind you you're worthy.

You deserve to have the body you love. And that can literally start now. Say it with me, "I AM WORTHY."

In the next chapter, I am excited to share with you the *relief* that could end your sabotaging ways for good. No longer will you experience start-again stop-again behaviors. The upcoming chapter will give you a new perspective to this journey. I'm excited for you to stay in this with me. Thank you for being here.

F.I.T. STRATEGY EXERCISE

The Funnel Effect

Below you will take part in a series of questions and answers.

— Step 1 —

Draw a funnel.

— Step 2 —

Pose this question at the top of the funnel: *What is my Eric?* In other words, what is your emotional weight? Why are you choosing to carry it around with you?

— Step 3 —

Answer the first question with a one sentence answer that is specific.

— Step 4 —

Next, restructure the answer into a new question. For example, if you answered, *I am holding on to childhood drama.* You would then ask yourself on the next line space, *Why am I holding on to childhood drama?* Continue this question and answer process until you get to a specific answer at the bottom of the funnel. You will have a better understanding of the reason for carrying the burden of emotional weight at the end of this process.

Structure each question with either *What* or *Why*.

Chapter 7

The Struggle is Where the Growth Is

*A stumbling block to the pessimist is a
stepping stone to the optimist.*

~ Eleanor Roosevelt

What is your greatest struggle when it comes to shedding pounds and being in shape?

Is it...

Self sabotage?

Your sweet tooth?

Lack of motivation to exercise?

Overeating?

A limiting self-belief?

We've talked about how imperative it is that you get why you do what you do. Certainly, understanding the deeper meaning to your underlying behaviors is the truth that shall set you free. In fact, in an ideal world, it would be awesome if you could be so painstakingly honest with yourself that you become enlightened on why you struggle with your body and then simply just fix it. But it's not as easy as just fixing it, is it?

More often than not, people find themselves struggling over and again with food and weight issues until they just give up. If you give up, I am telling you, you will miss the long-term reward completely. Because it is during your times of greatest struggle that you learn the most about yourself. It is in that struggle, where you can discover your greatest personal growths. Think back to a time in your life that was very complicated. Weren't there great lessons to be learned from that experience? And of course, you would have never moved into the experience had you known it would be difficult. But, knowing what you know now, you may even say that you are thankful for the experience, because you learned so much.

For many years, my struggle was going up and down on the scale. I would stay dedicated long enough to lose weight, but a couple of months or so of being at my ideal weight, I would begin to sabotage myself for a number of reasons. I would have the attitude that I could get away with it because I was skinnier. But it wasn't true. That was a lie that I told myself so that I could cheat. The truth was that I had not reconciled my internal feelings of self-doubt. I had not come to the point where I truly believed I could maintain my healthiest body. Even though my exterior looked different, the inside was still hurting and wanting to hold on to old behaviors. I ate for the wrong reasons, period. I was correct; I couldn't maintain a healthy body weight. Until I got to a place emotionally where I was willing to take a look at my struggle more intimately. I had to face my inner sabotagers, and grow through the experience. Let me rephrase that. I didn't have to. I chose to.

It is impossible to grow from success. You don't develop a skill, or gain confidence from the actual success. All of the development happens during the practice/training portion of the process. The success comes at the end, once all the work has been done. The real growth happens during the struggle. By definition, success means:

suc·cess

/sək'ses/

noun

1. the accomplishment of an aim or purpose.

It may be true that you've been spending so much of your time focused on how you're going to be successful at losing weight that you've missed the very components that will get you there which are: the lessons of the struggle. It's okay if the lessons seem hard. They are only hard because it's an area you haven't given focus.

It reminds me of learning to run a marathon. When I've run a marathon and come across the finish line with hands in the air, screaming, "Yaaaahoooo!!!" it is certainly a feeling of success. But I would not be able to claim that success if I had not struggled and fought through the last 26.2 miles of the race putting one foot in front of the other. It is in those quiet moments during the race that the internal struggle is at full force.

It's similar to the quiet moments in your car on the way home from work. When you are deciding to make food choices for your body that evening. Are you stressed and unconsciously going through the drive thru? Or are you conscious and mindfully deciding to give your body what it truly needs. Success is secured by what happens inside those moments. It is up to you to decide to let go of old patterns.

During my very first marathon, the Rock 'n' Roll San Diego Marathon, it suddenly became quite apparent to me that

I had been holding on to stuff from my past. Because I was at mile 22, I knew I was about to accomplish a HUGE GOAL for my life. I had never reached so far, or worked so hard for anything in my life, so the reality of knowing I would finish began to stir up an old stash of memories that I thought I had hidden. I was running along when I suddenly found myself completely overwhelmed with raw emotion. My eyes pooled up in tears, and I felt my throat tighten. I was moved with feelings of intensity. My mind flooded with all the times I had not followed through on a goal, felt regret, or disappointment in myself.

There I was, with people all around me running like horses to the barn. Some runners seemed intensely focused, and others seem to be desperately teetering between failure and success. I could hear their heavy breathing and moans. It was a heightened moment for me as I was silently experiencing my own kind of internal struggle. But it wasn't physical. I couldn't help but feel disappointed by things I had not completed in the past. Tears began to run down my face. I knew with every cell of my being that I wanted to be successful. Not just in that particular marathon, but in my life in general. In that moment, I decided NOT to carry the burdens of the past any further down the road. I made a pinky-swear-blood-bonding-to-the-end-of-my-days promise to myself. I swore to leave my disappointment in myself at mile 22.

Now because I'm a Hypnotist, I have trained myself to value and utilize metaphors and visions of the mind to create breakthroughs. This is something you can do too! Here's what I did. I visualized, as if it was real, a heaping pile of sludge drop off of me. It represented all that stuff that is no longer me. I heard Snoop Dog in my ears singing, "Drop it like it's hot, Drop it like it's hot." So I dropped it like it was hot alright and I never want to see it again. To this day it's somewhere between Genesee Avenue and Sea World Drive in San Diego, and I do not plan to ever go back and find it. Leaving it behind was a decision I made in mind. But it felt real, as if I could look back over my shoulder and actually see a big shitty pile of disappointment left on the race course. It's better there than in the back of my mind still influencing. Disappointment did not deserve to cross that finish line with me.

My truth came to the surface during my dire moment of struggle, and it became the catalyst for completing the race and feeling the success of crossing the finish line. Because of that experience, I will not disappoint myself again. I will always stand up to the challenge because I know the struggle will be worth my effort. You see, in striving to achieve your goal to getting healthy and maintaining it, you will be faced with obstacles. They will be in the form of self-doubt, a food choice, a decision to sleep in or go exercise. You can either cower at the obstacle and stay where you are, or you can choose to overcome it.

JOURNAL F.I.T. EXERICSE

Describe a moment or experience that seemed so difficult, yet you overcame it.

_____

_____

_____

_____

_____

_____

What is a truth you learned about yourself having experienced it?

_____

_____

_____

_____

_____

Based on that truth, what have you come to value greatly now?

_____

_____

_____

_____

_____

A SETBACK IS AN OPPORTUNITY FOR LEARNING

When we trip up in our healthy lifestyle program, we often refer to it as a setback. I'm sure you've heard yourself say it, "Well I was doing good, until I had a setback."

Let's chat about a hypothetical situation:

Julie was doing great on her weight loss plan, when one morning, she had a very stressful start to her day. The kids were not listening as they should. Their lack of timeliness got them all haphazardly out of the house, and late to school. A dude pulled out in front of her on the way to dropping off the kids, and it sent her stress level through the roof. The kids being late dominoed into Julie being late to work. Her supervisor was not happy about her tardiness and gave her a warning. The day felt like it was summing up to be a crappy one, and it had just started!

Then, right as Julie settled into her desk, along came a coworker friend with a box of glorious looking cinnamon rolls and scrumptious muffins. She thinks for a second, *No I shouldn't.* But she's stressed, and not in her conscious-thinking mind. Julie decides to give in to the temptation and splurge, thinking, *Screw it, my day is already messed up anyway!*

This is the classic scenario where triggering emotion triggers eating. Does this situation resonate with any of your personal experiences? With a strategic eye, you can instantly turn this setback into valuable insight that will allow success the next time around. If this happens to you, ask yourself *What, Why* and *How?*

What was I feeling?

What other factors were involved?

Why did I let myself fall for the trap?

How can I do better next time?

The purpose of asking yourself these questions is to understand the real reason for making the decision that you did. Take a moment to think about what is really going on in your head and emotions. Are you tempted to eat the goodies because you're hungry, or for another reason? Is it the imprint of a previous stress behavior?

Implore the F.I.T. Mindset and you will be able to take a step back from moments like the one described here. You'll be empowered to think about the key components of your stress and/or underlying emotions before committing to scarfing down a 600-calorie muffin and frappucino for reasons that don't really get fulfilled. Ralph Waldo Emerson says, "Our greatest glory is not in never failing, but in rising up every time we fail."

In actuality, when you truly do step back, you can use the opportunity to become clear. By learning from your setbacks, you are taking a stance in a more powerful position. When you take a step back to analyze and better understand the pitfalls you are repeatedly experiencing, you will be better equipped to handle the situation more positively the next time around.

There have been many Mind Body F.I.T. coaching calls

where one of the ladies confesses to splurging during our days apart. She comes to the call stricken with guilt and finds it hard to move on easily. I explain that guilt is a useless emotion when combined with food and indulging in it is very unproductive. What we can learn from a situation is much more empowering than wasting our energy on negative emotions. You can save yourself from feeling bad and spiraling into the internal abyss of your downfalls. It's a simple, old school method; learn from your mistakes.

I ask you ... How long does it take to eat a piece of chocolate cake? Eight or ten minutes? Eight to ten minutes of pure pleasure, right? The taste of the cake triggers off your receptors, and you feel good. You indulge and think, *Yum, this is incredible.*

Now answer this ... How long does fitting into a new sexy dress last? All evening long? Up to 300 minutes of pure confidence that can last beyond the strike of midnight! Or, knowing you have reached your goal body and are more fit than you have been in years? If you are awake from 6 a.m. to 10 p.m., that 'fit feeling' could last up to 16 hours or 960 minutes! There's no doubt that feeling good far outweighs the short term gratification.

Which is better, 8-10 minutes of pleasure from food? Or 960 minutes of confidence and heightened self-esteem, knowing that you followed through to your goal? To feel that feel-good feeling of knowing you are in the best shape of your life, you must be willing to make a decision in the moments of challenge. The struggle may be real. But it's a decision that ends the struggle. Next time the goodie box comes by, be strong enough to withstand your feelings of instant gratification.

Beware of the *Danger Signs!* If you recognize there is a lesson to be learned, and you choose not to learn it, you are deliberately resisting success. The resistance in itself is an opportunity to learn. Again, ask yourself the *What, why's* and *how's.*

What makes me resistant to change?

_____

_____

_____

_____

_____

_____

_____

How can I start doing better today?

_____

_____

_____

_____

_____

_____

_____

_____

It is imperative that you use your struggles to win your race. View them as an opportunity to know who you are. There is no such thing as failure if you always transform your challenge into a lesson. Brian Tracy says, "Never consider the possibility of failure; as long as you persist, you will be successful."

MOVING INTO ACTION

There is no need to beat yourself up in the future. From here on out, you will be utilizing your inner mind to release weight. All the facets of your character, your mind-body communication, and your personal belief systems will be the strength you need to accomplish your goals. I will teach you a secret weapon in the next chapter that will propel you to your goals. This could be life transforming ... let's go! *Push Past Limitations.* View a mistake as an opportunity to learn and forgive yourself.

F.I.T. STRATEGY EXERCISE

The Struggle is Where the Growth Is

Recall two specific experiences where your weight struggle has given you the gift of learning and growing. Place your hand on your heart. Close down your eyes. Slowly inhale and exhale five deep breaths, whispering the words, "Relax and Recall," with each inhalation and exhalation. With pencil and paper in front of you, journal your answer (or write straight into this book). Ask your inner thoughts to flow from your mind and onto the paper providing you valuable insight.

What have I learned from my weight struggle?

_____

_____

_____

_____

_____

_____

What have I made it mean about me, that it doesn't have to?

_____

_____

_____

_____

_____

_____

Chapter 8

Observe Your Thinking Patterns

If you hear a voice within you saying,
'You are not a painter,' then by all means
paint and that voice will be silenced.

~ Vincent Van Gogh

Let's examine the relationships in your life. Are you a good friend to your best girlfriend? Do you listen, give positive feedback and encourage? Do you tell her she's beautiful when she's feeling bad that her favorite pants don't fit? Do you give her constructive feedback when she asks for it? You will often go to the ends of the earth for your closest friend. If she needs you, you are there as support. No matter what, you are prepared to celebrate with her or give her a pep talk if need be. I am asking you to do the same for yourself. Through this health journey, learn to be your own best friend. Treat yourself with the same love and kindness that you have shown to others. Isn't it interesting? When you screw up, you are so quick to judge yourself and slam yourself for your mistakes. Yet, if it was a friend in that position, you would give them plenty of reasons why they didn't mess up so bad. You would be the voice of optimism and offer up a biased perspective.

When life serves up a meltdown, don't head for your comfort food. Instead, learn to rally up your best friend spirit to pick up the pieces. Infuse your daily life with the same synergistic quality you receive when you get together with a friend. Utilize a journal to share, express, laugh or cry. Check in with yourself, just like your best friend would. When this 'soul searching' approach to shedding extra pound uncovers fear or sadness inside of you, seek forgiveness, healing and letting go. Embrace your body and work on it, rather than complain or stay powerless. Be the person you would want to hang out with that is inspiring.

The great business and life philosopher Jim Rohn says, "To be attractive you must become attractive." My interpretation of that quote is, you must work on yourself. People like positive people. When is the last time you enjoyed hanging around a grump? That's no fun, is it? It is unfair to yourself to spend days on end in a slouch mood just because you had a week that felt disastrous.

Resilience is an important part of winning the weight challenge. You can't wait for someone to complain to about your week or hope that your girlfriend calls so that you can go on about the fact that you are a loser because you ate a hamburger and fries. You have to be the one that plays the part of the best friend, and say to yourself, *You are not a loser, you had a learning experience. What was the difference between how it made you feel psychologically versus how it made your body feel? How can you move forward, and when do you start?*

Be the quintessential BFF; listen to your heart, connect with your spirit, cheer yourself up and move forward. This method for weight loss is not about one day in your life; it's about the journey.

A friend once told me she was always disappointed with her birthdays. For more than forty years she would anticipate the day and was continually disappointed that no one would offer to take her to dinner, send a card, or even wish her a *Happy Birthday.* She decided that she was tired of feeling bad year after year, and it was time for the pity party to be over. So she took matters into her own hands and made an agreement with herself. Every birthday, she calls the flower shop and orders the most gorgeous bouquet they have, with the delivery note signed to: The Birthday Girl. When the flowers are delivered to her door, she says it puts a smile on her face and joy in her heart.

When you take care of yourself, it motivates you to take even better care of yourself. As a self-assured woman, do not judge your value based on someone else's opinions or actions. You take matters into your own hands and create the life you desire. Those that truly love you will support you in your confidence and uphold you for your strength.

What if you are accustomed to beating yourself up and don't know how to be your own friend?

It has long been recorded by the great leaders of our time that positive self-talk must be practiced to create personal success. I had not learned of this process until I was nearly thirty years old. It was while attending Hypnotherapy training that I was introduced to the concept of positive self-talk, and I quickly became enamored with the methods. Up until that time, I was accustomed to beating myself up with brutal internal language. My thoughts were often negative, and I consistently talked myself out of potentially positive situations. I can recall many pinnacle moments where an opportunity came my way, and because I had very little self-value, I would pass the opportunity by. These thinking habits did not just develop all on their own. They were learned.

I was raised in an environment where Mom regularly criticized Dad. She was resentful of the choices he made to leave their marriage and in reflection, it felt like I spent more than half my childhood defending Dad's character. It drove me and my sister crazy. Her goal to make us dislike our Dad backfired however. We were so tired, annoyed and frustrated by what seemed like continuous, totally off base accusations that we began to be critical of her, instead of him. Mom trained me to be a critical and argumentative person. She modeled it and this critical nature became my way, that is, until I learned a new way much later in life. This is not about blame as I have forgiven her (and I suggest you do the same if you have a parent like this), but it is about recognizing the pattern. Awareness will shed light on the pattern, but you also must take action in changing it. Actually DO something beneficial with your awareness. (That's why I'm writing this book!)

When I was 17 years old, I begged Mom to send me to John Robert Powers Modeling School. I had hopes that they could teach me the skills I needed to know to launch a modeling career. Even though I dreamt of being in the spotlight, I had not developed confidence or real talent to back it up. Mom obliged, and modeling school lasted about eight months. We learned makeup application, runway modeling and how to pose for print work. It was fun and gave me the feeling that I was on my way to super stardom. To the external world it seemed that I was progressing nicely, but I had many internal struggles that I was dealing with; the pain of being in the middle of two parents who hated one another, school social issues and a constant battle with my body. I was always on a diet. I believed I had to look a certain way to be accepted.

One day John Robert Powers called me in for an audition. They were auditioning about 200 girls, searching for the prototypical "California Bikini Girl" as they called it, for an upcoming commercial magazine advertisement. The job was for a business by the name of 98 Degrees, a swimwear company out of Orange County, CA. After going through the auditions, I got a callback. They wanted me to come in for round two of the model search. They had me model one of their bikinis and shoot some photos. Much to my surprise, at the end of the second audition, they informed me I had won the part. I was ecstatic! While standing there excited about the news that I was their chosen girl, they went on to inform me the details of the upcoming shoot. The woman said, "Please be at such and such address next Saturday at 7 a.m. in Newport Beach and try to drop five or ten pounds this week. Okay, great, thank you. See you next Saturday."

I had a silent conniption in my head. Stunned, I hesitantly half-smiled and said, "Thank You." I left the studio, and headed for home freaking out! I thought, *Holy crud, I have to lose five or ten pounds by next week?* Body struggles were already a recurring issue for me, and now my body image was being judged in public, and I felt my future was on the line. I felt so much pressure that all I could do was what I had always relied on in troubled times—EAT!

I ate my way through the week with bakery items of every kind. As I ate to self-soothe, I became more and more stressed that I couldn't stop myself from eating. The feelings of guilt soon set in, but I was debilitated to do anything about it. As I sabotaged myself with food, my internal thoughts were destructive and cruel:

You're not worthy of being a model anyway.

You Suck!

You're Ugly!

My inner language wasn't pretty. I do believe the request to lose five or ten pounds in a week was too much to ask of a teenager, or anyone for that matter. It was a very unrealistic demand. Thankfully, our world has come a long way with body positivity and what healthy looks like. Nevertheless, on that day, what really fueled my self-sabotaging behavior was the practice of negative self-talk. I backed out of the job, and the 2nd runner up that was thinner and more beautiful than me (or so I thought) completed the shoot.

When I later learned the processes of positive self-talk, many experiences like the one described here came rushing to my mind. I felt sad thinking about all the times I had wasted energy on feeling unworthy. But that's because I had put so much emphasis on external beauty. That's why it is vital that you and I explore ourselves and abandon old self-ideals. Most often they were built upon a throne of lies anyhow. You don't want to recycle that stuff!

One day back in Hypnotherapy training, while studying limiting belief behaviors, I said to my instructor, "So what you're saying is, be aware of what you say, because your mind is always listening." He replied, "Yes, listening and recording." That thought has stuck with me ever since.

"Be aware of what you say, because your mind is always listening."

I continue to say it to myself as a reminder to keep my thoughts focused on what I want, instead of what I don't want. Michael Singer, author of one of my favorite books, The Untethered Soul, says, "There is nothing more important to true growth than realizing that you are not the voice of the mind, you are the one who hears it."

It's so true. Our thoughts are powerful; they are the seeds that compose our internal beliefs about ourselves. If we water and cultivate our thoughts, they will grow into actions and sprout into a tangible, physical reality. Advances in neuroscience prove the progression of thinking habits, and the high degree of influence they have on our bodies.

Make Optimism Your Oxygen

Guaranteed, your world will change. John Addison, an accomplished composer and Academy Award winner says, "You've got to win in your mind before you win in your life." We must be scrupulous in the thoughts we choose. Not to the point of anxiety, but to mindfully learn a practice. Our thoughts, positive or negative, will create a result, guaranteed.

Our minds are resourceful and without conscious awareness, we automatically seek personal rightness.

That means we gravitate towards an outcome that proves ourselves right. Just like I did in the 17-year-old modeling job, I believed I was not worthy of the part, and I proved myself right. The outcome gave me a reason to say to myself, *See, I told you. You could never be a model.*

Self-defeating thinking is toxic to your goals, and aspirations. If you had a gallon of clear water in a bucket, and you dropped in just one ounce of white paint, your water would become clouded, infiltrating the clarity of the other one hundred twenty-seven ounces. Just like the paint creating a visual result in the water, negative, sabotaging thoughts hinder your success and muddy up your vision of what is possible for you.

Your mind is constantly, unconsciously talking to your body. We know it as Mind-Body Communication. We are going to take the quote I shared with you, *"Be aware of what you say, because your mind is always listening,"* and kick it up a notch. *"Be aware of what your mind is thinking, because your body is receiving."*

You are Responsible for the Physical Shape Your Body is In

The quote above should drive the point home, big time! Read it again. You have more control than you might realize. Your mind is absolutely creating your physical results. As you learned in Chapter 3, the power to make living healthy easy comes from your subconscious mind. Your stored thoughts, feelings and experiences are creating the body you have now.

Everything you say and do is being recorded by all levels

of your consciousness. Physical, mental, emotional, spiritual, and even at a cellular level; your mind is always archiving your thoughts and actions. One of the most famous stories I know of mind-body healing is from author and spiritual leader Louise Hay. In her book *You Can Heal Your Body* she shares her story of healing herself from cancer in the 1980s through the use of powerful affirmations. Her experiment on herself and the positive result, inspired her to write the book and develop an entire glossary of physical ailments that can be healed or dissolved through affirmative thought.

The mind-body-spirit is an intense relationship intricately connected as one. How is it that you can produce real, physical tears from simply watching a movie that is a rehearsed scene of two people you don't even know? It's because your mind-body-spirit are linked. You are emotionally invested in an image, thought or idea. There is just no denying its power. It's truly amazing that you can make yourself physically sick from mental worry, literally having to vomit from a life situation that you are struggling with or break out in hives from stress. Your mind and emotions are powerful and are truly the control panel for your body.

Many people think the mind-body conversation is spiritual talk as if it's a belief just for the yoga and metaphysical groups. The mind and body connection is not a belief. It's a fact. Your mind has been in your body since your birth. It's how you've done everything! Every growth experience you've ever had has been a combination of unison learning between your mind and body. Every book your mind has read, your body was present and paying attention in silence. Every physical experience, traumatic and victorious, your mind took notes in the background.

Engage your mind and emotions to output a new physical result. You've been so focused on just what you put into your mouth. It's not totally about the food. Now you can rejoice that you know how to take command! Let's take a look at how your inner mind relates to food. Everything we think is in pictures or knowingness. If I ask you to think of an apple, it may suddenly flash on the screen of your mind. It's even in vivid detail. Do it right now. Think of an apple—you can instantly describe the color, the shape and the texture. If I said, "Don't think of that apple anymore," you couldn't help but continue to think about the apple.

If I say, "Don't think of your favorite ice cream!" Suddenly that flavor ice cream flashes into your mind. It may be a cone, a cup, chocolate chip or rainbow; your mind creates an image of an ice cream whether I told you to think of an ice cream, or not to. When you are trying to eat only healthy foods, and you have told yourself that you CANNOT have snacks and CANNOT have desert, all you find yourself thinking about is what you CANNOT have. It has nothing to do with your willpower or your ability to stick with a program. Just like the ice cream, you envisioned the ice cream even though I told you NOT to. It's just a simple fact of how your mind operates.

Make a promise to yourself that you will no longer deprive yourself from certain foods, and you'll utilize the mechanisms of your mind more purposefully. The real power comes from knowing that all foods are a CHOICE. You are creating a lifestyle. There is no beginning and end like the old Fat Mindset. You are empowered with a F.I.T. Mindset and it is how you live, making the beneficial food choices that provide you energy and health and allow you to live in a body you value and respect. You do this while also enjoying chocolate, chips or whatever, in appropriate amounts at appropriate times. It wasn't that one small handful that created the issue. It was the consistency for all the wrong reasons.

LET'S TALK BODY IMAGE

Breaking it down more simply, body (meaning physical) and image (mind, pictures, visualizations) are essentially what and how you think about your body. The same association principals apply. If you are constantly thinking about how much you DO NOT like the size of your butt or your gut, you will just get more of the same, dislike towards that body part. Negating certain parts of your body is an unhealthy practice. Have you said, "Hey Fatty!" while catching a glimpse in the mirror when you step out of the shower? Have you cursed your stomach while trying to zip up your too-small jeans? Or the opposite; you avoid looking in the mirror altogether. What's the internal message you're still sending? That type of thinking stops here.

We once did a positive-body-parts challenge within our Mind Body F.I.T. Group. The ladies were asked to post pictures in our private Facebook group of body parts they are choosing to wholeheartedly embrace. The goal was to curb them from thinking negatively to highlighting parts of their body they can love and appreciate. One posted a close-up of her lips touting her fondness for the fullness and shape. Another appreciated her feet and legs for all the places she had ventured. The challenge went joyfully on with hands for hard work, and boobs for breastfeeding. One morning I tapped the group link and was immediately faced with a picture of a naked butt as our brave and outgoing Sara B. showcased how much she loved her latina backside. HaHa! I love it.

It's impossible to trade your body in for another, so it's high time that you embrace all of you and begin anew. To create your best health, you must accept where you're at, focus on being positive about your parts, and build from there. Because your mind thinks in pictures, and your subconscious is vast, imagine how much you could influence your good by recruiting your innate, creative abilities, and apply them to your physical goals. Don't underestimate the power of a repeated affirmation.

"I am learning to accept, nurture and love my body by eating well and moving more."

The goal is to focus on being a good leader to yourself. Constantly trying to control your thoughts and eating choices can be stressful. So instead of controlling, I suggest you loosen the reins just a tad and focus on management. A good manager is a person who listens, collaborates and is focused on solutions.

In a recent Forbes article showcasing traits of an excellent manager and leader, the author gathered evidence to hone in on seven specific skill sets they tend to possess.

1. *They Love the Company Culture.*
2. *They're Positively Contagious.*
3. *They Can Sustain Focus.*
4. *They Lead With Their Head and Heart.*
5. *They're Honest.*
6. *They Take Accountability.*
7. *They're Effective at Making Decisions.*

Imagine the progress you can make in your self-care by adopting this type of thinking and internal communication.

1. *You create your internal culture.*
2. *Your positivity is contagious.*
3. *You learn to sustain focus.*
4. *You lead your self care choices with head and heart.*
5. *You are honest with yourself.*
6. *You take personal accountability.*
7. *You are effective in making decisions.*

Your role is to lead your life with health and vitality by the decisions you make. Think of your body as a ship and your mind as the captain. As the person in charge, you have full authority of what cargo and crew goes on and off your ship. Just like life circumstances, you do not have control over the weather, but you can determine what direction you can maneuver around it or strategize how to get through it with victory.

Your co-worker is going to get sick and leave you with a ton of work, your garage will unexpectedly flood and your cousin's big party wedding will throw you off your health focus for a couple of days. None of these circumstances need to send you into an eating binge or lack of exercise for days on end. Lead your life with the mindset of health, and it'll be who you are every day, despite circumstances.

THE FREEDOM MODEL

Begin to practice good listening skills. Listen to what your mind is thinking, and what your mouth is saying. This is neuroscience in action! Recognize that you are not your thoughts, you are the observer of your thoughts. The best way to begin creating space in your overthinking is observance. Realizing that you have the ability to step out of your thoughts is a passage to peace.

Once you learn to observe repeated unbeneficial thoughts (worry, fear, self-doubt), it's like stepping off a perpetual "mind merry-go-round". You may be shocked at how often you insult yourself or contradict your abilities in this fitness realm. You cannot feel good about who you are becoming if your mind is poisonously repeating self-defeating thoughts. Employ the Freedom Model and it will help you create **A.R.T.** with your thoughts and emotions.

A.R.T. ACRONYM

Awareness. Release. Trust.

You are in need of every tool you've got to overcome that part of you that often gets in the way of your own health-success. These three steps practiced mindfully and intentionally will be your artful force within. Like Luke from Star Wars. Luke says, "I can't believe it." Yoda answers, "And this is why you fail." You are either believing in the power of the force or negating you possess it.

Believe in your power within to decipher your path. Your thoughts, if given self-defeating power, can lead you down the road of fear, anger, grief and self-loathing. There is so much darkness there, it could take hours, days or even months to realize you need to turn the light on. Yet, this freedom model will deepen your emotional intelligence. It is the bridge of courage. In his amazing book *Letting Go, the Pathway to Surrender* by David Hawkins, he shares his research on the measures of the emotional scale. The emotion of courage is the very gift you can give yourself, to release from the pull of heavy emotional burdens. When you choose courage, you are choosing to embody an energy that neutralizes darkness and allows you to release it.

THE STEPS IN THE FREEDOM MODEL ARE TO FIRST OBSERVE YOUR THOUGHTS AND EMOTIONS

— Step 1 —

Awareness

Step out and be objective. You can do this by imagining the process in your mind, or by both imagining it and physically doing it. See, feel, know and practice stepping out of the chaos of your thinking and into a perspective of observance. Like the saying, "You can't see the forest for the trees." When you step out, you can broaden your perspective and shift what you focus on.

— Step 2 —

Release

Release what does not serve your highest good and refocus on what does. We so often hold on to things much longer than we need to. Things people say to us, situations that do not go as planned, the many that we fail, life circumstances we deem unfair, the list is endless. The longer or more intensely you hold on, will determine the length of your suffering.

To successfully release, it may look like forgiving (yourself or others). It may look like surrendering. Each time you choose to engage in this freedom model, it will require some form of letting go of the need to control the outcome, or the need for the result to be in your favor. Know that letting go is always in your favor. Your internal dysfunctional needs are often running the show unconsciously, and that is not who or what you want directing your life. Let go and trust.

— Step 3 —
Trust

To truly trust oneself, is to trust the universal spirit of all things. You may call that God. As it states in the Bible, "You are in me and I am in you." For many, it is a deep sense of truth, a knowingness, a universal force. In psychological, humanistic terms, we can define self-trust as a deep sense of self-reliance, knowing that no one can be as supportive to you as you can be to yourself. It is trust that helps you build self-confidence in decision making, and the ability to handle the pressures of life in more meaningful and thoughtful ways without sacrificing your health.

Practice linking together these three steps of awareness, release and trust, making it a thinking habit that you can apply in practical ways.You'll find that this practice has a myriad of helpful benefits. In your food choices you'll be able to step back and make a clear decision for your health. You'll be able to recognize when you're about to inhale a bag of chips, and actually make a choice that serves both immediate and long term needs. You'll learn to trust and love yourself more. You'll also fine-tune your ability to de-stress in more beneficial ways, or create space in difficult relationships that need boundaries or forgiveness. You'll discover that with this practice, you'll need less turning to vices for temporary fulfillment, and you'll get more of actually meeting your emotional needs.

Because positive self-talk and the Freedom Model practice happens only within you, no one needs to know what you're thinking or doing. It can be implemented any time, any day, anywhere. There is no limit to its effectiveness, and cannot be overused. With your thoughts, your Freedom Model can transform your attitude, and help you strengthen your courage to take a stand, make a good decision or get through a difficult moment. Even if you don't fully believe in your ability to create a shift right now, trust that repetition will begin to take hold, and you will soon believe. So...get busy practicing!

F.I.T. EXERCISE: THE FREEDOM MODEL

Close your eyes. Place your hand on your heart. Inhale and exhale several purposeful breaths. With each breath whisper, "I let go of grievances and choose the miracle." *Ask yourself ...*

Awareness: What is one thing I've been holding on to for way too long? What is one thing I keep overthinking?

_____

_____

_____

_____

Release: Who or what do I need to forgive to truly let it go? Myself? The situation?

_____

_____

_____

_____

Trust: In what ways can I now shift from looking outside for answers, and instead look within and trust myself to know, do and be?

_____

_____

_____

_____

Bridge Phrases: How to create affirmations that actually work.

When you are tempted to succumb to a food craving, you can draw from your secret weapon with a positive self-affirming thought, *I am managing my mind better, and focused on long-term gratification.*

Next time you're at the grocery store and you smell the fresh baked bread from the bakery oven, your mind may say, *I am dedicated to my lifestyle plan, and love myself for my commitment.*

During a social gathering, while others are indulging in a platter of cheesy bread and potato skins, your mind says, *I stick to my plan of hovering at the veggie platter, and I am happy about my empowered choice.*

Positive Affirmations/Self-Talk can be easily utilized to help you reach success, and for many different weight loss obstructions.

Warning: Do not underestimate the power of reframing your thoughts. Your internal thoughts are robust and mighty! Utilize them to be your springboard towards achieving your goals. "It's the repetition of affirmations that leads to belief. And once that belief becomes a deep conviction, things begin to happen," said Claude M. Bristol. Focus on cultivating supportive, loving thoughts.

So what happens when ... ? You look in the mirror, say the magic words with conviction, and hear your inner mind say after your beautiful affirmation... "I am my ideal weight and I love my body ... bullshit, bullshit, bullshit."

What happens then? Do you say, "Affirmations don't work"? You're right. They don't work when you don't believe them from the get-go. I have a solution for that!

As a professional Hypnotist, I am quite skilled at talking to the mind, knowing your cognitive brain is listening, as well as your subconscious. I created a brain hack called *Magic Mindset: How to Get Your Affirmations to Actually Work.*

The secret to getting your affirmations to work is threefold.

1. Add Emotion
2. Use Bridge Phrases
3. Repetition

Bridge words placed in your affirmation make them believable. Your subconscious mind is irrational, emotional and repetitive. Therefore, it is your opportunity to take advantage of those attributes.

Try it. Transform the above affirmation from ... "I am my ideal weight and I love my body" to "I am in the process of being my ideal weight and I am learning to love my body." Now, say it again, and this time with confidence!

"I am in the process of being my ideal weight and I am learning to love my body."

You can say it and believe it! It also prompts you to make a better choice next time you are eating, or reframe the way you talk to yourself when you're putting on your pants.

Valuable Bridge Phrases

"I am ...

"In the process of ..."
"Learning ..."
"Choosing ..."

Here are just a few ideas.
Utilize when...

- Looking at your body in the mirror. *"I am learning to love and embrace me!"*

- Pushing through a strenuous moment while exercising. *"I can do it, I am learning I am stronger than I realize!"*

- You feel defeated. *"I am learning to be resilient and believe in myself."*

- Feeling tempted to binge. *"I am learning how to be in control and am choosing to win."*

- Your boss is reprimanding you. *"I am open to learning."*

- You've made a poor food choice. *"I forgive myself and am learning that food matters."*

- Before an interview, a sale, or an important meeting. *"I bring value and excellence to all that I do."*

- Communicating with a loved one. *"I am learning to love myself, and choose to receive love as well."*

- Dealing with a difficult client. *"I am choosing to be patient and kind."*

- Having a challenging day. *"I am happy to learn from every situation."*

- Another driver cuts you off. *"I choose to respond with love and kindness."*

- A co-worker tempts you with the candy bowl. *"I am in control of my choices."*

- The vending machine is calling your name. *"I recognize temptation, and value my strength to say no."*

- Your clothes don't quite fit. *"I persevere knowing I shall overcome."*

- You're fearful. *"I am choosing to have courage."*

- You're filled with self-doubt. *"Every day I am learning ways that I am more capable."*

At the end of the chapter you can create affirmations of your own and integrate them into your daily life. I encourage you to put them into your digital calendar on your phone and set them to pop up first thing in the morning and night. Let them be the last thing you read before you drift off to sleep, and the first thing you read to start your day.

This strategy can really work for you, when you actually do it. Hundreds upon thousands of times, my positive self-talk has pushed me through to success. I can recall many times running up a hill in the mountains of Lake Arrowhead, and feeling so challenged that I wanted to quit. If I start to hear myself thinking, *I feel like I'm going to keel over,* I instantly replace the thought with, *Delete, Delete! I am choosing to be strong, I am powerful, I've got this!* Because I know the power of my thoughts, I choose to fill my mind with only positive internal language. When I am feeling weak at the end of a marathon, I go completely internal. I think to myself, *You can do this De'Anna, Come On, Dig. You got This!*

It may even be as simple as a favorite food calling my name from the kitchen. I think, *Nope, you're not part of my plan. I am more important than eating you.*

Following through in completing written affirmations will be a stepping stone to your health goals. As you begin to train your mind to think in this manner, you'll be able to create them instantly and apply them anytime you need them ... they are your *Mindset Magic.*

SAY THANK YOU AND BELIEVE IT

You now have your mind moving in the direction of your goals; it's time to implore your secret weapon in accepting a compliment. I always think it's sad when women find it difficult to truly acknowledge a compliment. When you have given your friend a compliment, and she gives you every reason why your compliment is not true, it's disappointing. After all, you gave the compliment because you meant it. You voiced your thoughts because you felt it was important to say.

SPEAK POSITIVELY TO YOUR CURVES!

It's a true telling sign about how a woman feels on the inside when she can't accept a compliment. Own your beauty and presence. Resist the temptation to point out your flaws. As you continue your weight release transformation, hold your shoulders back, carry yourself with confidence, and practice positive self-talk. Be gracious when accepting a compliment and believe it's true. Receive the compliment like a gift for your ever-growing self-esteem.

When someone says, "You look great, you've lost weight haven't you?" Be sincere, and say, "Thanks I've been taking care of myself." You are simply being honest and appreciative. When you accept a compliment, remember, your subconscious is recording data. You want your unconscious mind to hear you!

Equipped with your *Mindset Magic*, you are now ready to take it to the next level in Chapter 9.

Get ready my friend, the next chapter is sure to be a wild ride that will challenge you to step up. You may find yourself screaming like you're on a crazy amusement park ride, because I'm going to ask you to start stepping out of your comfort zone. Have no worries, it will be fun, and my strategy promises you may never be the same woman again ... you'll be better. Say it with me, "I can do it. I am strong!"

F.I.T. STRATEGY EXERCISE

My BFF

Journal a list of affirmations that represent the new seeds you are choosing to plant in your mind. Write 10-20 of them for this fruitful exercise.

Tip! A positive affirmation is always written in the form of "NOW," as if you have it already. For example, the incorrect form is, "I want to feel more worthy." The correct form is, "I AM WORTHY." Notice how empowering the "I AM" affirmation is compared to the other?

Remember, you are feeding your mind, and with repetition, will override the old self-defeating thoughts. Choose to feed yourself encouraging, loving words that will be watered, cultivated and will sprout a tangible result.

Utilize the Bridge Phrases to Make Them Believable When Necessary

"I am ...

"*In the process of ...*"

"*Learning ...*"

"*Choosing ...*"

Lastly, transfer these affirmations to your digital calendar on your phone and set a reminder for them to pop up at bedtime and again in the morning. Read them with emotion morning and night, as if you are seeding your inner *mindfull garden.*

1 _____

2 _____

3 _____

4 _____

5 _____

6 _____

7 _____

8 _____

9 _____

10 _____

11 _____

12 _____

13 _____

14 _____

15 _____

PART 3

THE HEROINE TAKES ACTION

Chapter 9

Courageous Active Faith

Be the heroine of your own story. Swoop in
and empower the powerless parts of you.

~ De'Anna Nunez

We've talked a lot about the built-in tool of repetition within your subconscious mind. New repeated actions that are outside of your old norm will create habits and beliefs that will propel you to your goals. In order to do that, you must create an abrupt shift in your patterns. It's called a **pattern interrupt**. I first heard this term studying *Humanistic Neuro Linguistic Programming* from my amazing mentor Gary DeRodriguez. It carries a big importance in my Coaching and Hypnotherapy work.

A pattern interrupt is a way to change your mental state or underlying behavior strategy. Your habit patterns are a behavior sequence or a neural pathway. At any point, you can choose to disrupt that sequence and start anew. When you are spiraling into a psychological rabbit hole, about to snack yourself off track from your health goals, you can perform a pattern interrupt.

It can be as easy as:

- Go for a walk
- Reach out to a friend
- Check in with your community support (Mind Body F.I.T. Club ladies are awesome with this)
- Put the food away
- Watch something humorous
- Check in with your journal or written goals

PATTERN INTERRUPTS
EXTERNAL TIPS TO THRIVE

Essential oils perform an olfactory pattern interrupt. Our five senses are connected to our subconscious mind. You recall memories, positive and negative through vision, hearing, smell, taste and touch. You are also recording everything you do now through those senses. Have you ever thought about your favorite food and when you get so encaptured by the thought it's as if you can smell it or taste it?

Essential oils are a fun way to interrupt unconscious patterns. Lemon is a gentle boost for mental clarity, as well as black pepper, lavandin, spearmint, rosemary, cedarwood, eucalyptus and basil. Simply open the bottle and breathe in the scent. You can also use a diffuser or dilute with a carrier oil such as coconut or almond oil on your skin.

THE RISE WITH HYPNOKINESTHETICS

A book, *Healing with HypnoKinesthetics,* by my colleague Patrica Vessey has been particularly helpful to my coaching clients. Among all her great suggestions and insights, her mind-body poses are a standout for a method of pattern interrupt. When you are feeling any kind of stress - anxiety, uncertainty, powerless or angry, perform this pose pattern interrupt. I took her pose and put my own Mind Body F.I.T. spin on it.

Instructions:

Pose 1: Interpret what you are feeling (overwhelm, sadness, anger, etc) by embodying a physical pose that symbolizes the feeling. By doing so you are acknowledging the feeling versus suppressing or projecting.

Pose 2: Transition into pose 2 by saying, "Rise like I've risen before." Interpret your "rise feeling" by embodying a physical pose that symbolizes the feeling of rise. Transition into Pose 3, from "the rise."

Pose 3: Interpret the feeling of "power" by embodying a physical pose that symbolizes the feeling of power.

In each pose, close your eyes, experience the feeling inside your body. Become in tune with that feeling and open yourself up to acceptance of the feeling. Now, in a flow-fashion, shift from one pose to the next. Feel the feeling, accept the feeling and flow through it, shifting from one to the next. Repeat the whole 1-3 pose pattern 7-10 times. You'll notice in a matter of minutes, your initial entrapped emotion is interrupted with a feeling of empowerment.

Studies in neuroscience show us how flexible our neuropathways are. It's just not true that people can't change. Perhaps the ones that perpetuate that idea are the people who are resistant to change? You, however, are embracing it.

Are your goals aligned with the evolved woman you see as your future self? Or, are you misaligned and staying within your comfort zone?

Change doesn't happen in your current comfort zone. Yet that is where you spend most of your time! It's for that very reason, you must have the courage to recognize when your place of comfort needs upgrading, because there is joy and possibilities awaiting you in doing things differently. Imagine the shift that will occur as you let new ideas, concepts, and ways of being into your comfort zone. It can't possibly remain the same!

It is human to desire predictability. Our schedules and routines create the safety we seek. We get up at the same time each day, we run off to work, we check our phone and email. When something messes with our schedule, we get thrown off. We think we need that predictability in our lives. Our homes for example; we have our favorite chair. We sit in the same place at the dining table. We drink our coffee or tea out of the same cup. We sleep in the same position in our beds. We tend to rotate the same foods in our meals, all because it's our programmed experience. It comforts us to know what to expect. But it's the unexpected things in life that often bring us our greatest joy!

Answer me this, how often do new, experiential things happen inside your house? Hardly ever. Just about everything you experience happens outside your home. Sure, books you read and access to the Internet have an influence on you, but truly, you could be inside your home and experience very little that is new. It could remain, for the most part, an extremely predictable environment. Where is the adventure in that? Let's discuss all the reasons why you want to expand your comfort zone.

Your current comfort zone is ...

- Familiar

- Routine

- Typical

- Constant

- Programmed

- Expected

Are your goals, the evolved woman you see as your future, inside that comfort zone? *Nope!? Or Yes!?*

If you stay believing and doing the same things about yourself, you will receive the same predictable results. Knowing what to expect provides personal security even when you're expecting the mundane, the dysfunctional or even abuse. You are phenomenal at adaptation. But let's be clear, you must keep your finger on the pulse of what you are adapting to and assure it is aligned with your greater good. In order to break out of the habits and beliefs you've settled into, you must be willing to think new things. You are now stepping out of the familiar and into the unknown. There is great reward to be had by accepting this invitation to leap with faith into the new you. I call it ... Courageous Active Faith.

I had a woman bravely share on a coaching call one evening, her realization that for years she had been letting other people control her life. She had been living as the quintessential nice girl for so long that she hardly stood up for herself anymore. She had little personal identity. She just took on the emotional crap of others and kept burying her resentment. She had used food as her self-soothing mechanism. It wasn't until she chose to have courage, looking within for strength, that she uncovered her limiting factor and created a breakthrough.

With another woman, Lynda, we worked on the fear of her father in a Hypnosis session. She felt she had created a real mental block surrounding the abuse she endured as a kid, and she knew it was holding her back. At this time of her life, in her fifties, she was on a crusade to push through all her fears and so we did a breakthrough session. I used a technique to shift her subconscious and it was as if she came out of hiding. She said as a result of the session, she could finally stop thinking of her father as a monster and have compassion for what he was going through. Lynda went on to write a book called *The Year of Fears* where she talks about facing a fear every day for a year. Her confidence grew immensely, and she now leads many other women to overcome their fears.

Fear begins in the brain and sends messages to your body. It can be real or imagined, it doesn't matter, your mind and body respond regardless. When you become instantly frightened by a person, thing or situation, you immediately react based on your internal survival system in the brain. Your amygdala kicks in and you have a fight, flight (or freak out) response. My husband loves to scare me and thinks it's hysterical. I swear, one of these times he's going to get punched in the face! You know the feeling, as if your whole body goes into high alert like a cartoon character with eyes bulging and hair standing on end. What you are really feeling is your brain releasing chemicals into the body, and that's when you feel the sensations of your heart racing, shortness of breath, and a reactiveness you are not consciously controlling. You know that feeling! It takes a few minutes to calm yourself down.

Fear can also be experienced without any outside circumstances happening. It is entirely created in your mind! When you feel that kind of fear, it hits your senses and your stomach flutters, heart pounds, blood pressure can rise, tightness in the throat, some people break out in hives or even vomit. I point out this phenomenal reactive mechanism because it demonstrates to you the incredible connection between your mind, imagination and body. You actually have total control over that, but most people don't take the time to learn how.

I shared with you that I've overcome extreme stage fright. I did that by using Self-Hypnosis. I focused inward and targeted the sensations in my body with a new message attached. I told myself to interpret those feelings in my stomach as excitement. I'd love for you to start practicing this awareness too. Here is an example of what you'd hear if you were inside my mind before an important speaking presentation. My hope in sharing this with you, is to give you some ideas on how you can reframe your thoughts and create new interpretations of mind and body.

INSIDE MY HEAD BACKSTAGE

De'Anna, hey girl, those flips flops in your stomach? They're telling you something amazing is about to happen. This isn't just any old day on the couch. This is an opportunity that can change your life and someone else's too. You are now breathing with ease, deep breaths, calming down any nerves to a more, gentle sensation. It's okay to be scared. It's a good thing. Something exciting is happening! God, Universe and all that is love, speak through me, guide my words and touch someone today who is here to hear what they need to hear. You are alive and this moment is meant to be, because you were chosen for this experience. Settle in, you got this.

I encourage you to see this process for what it is. It is not just positive thinking, it's commanding your mind and telling your subconscious what you expect. You can get better at deciphering when you have real fear, and when it's created fear. One is necessary and there to serve you and protect you. The other type of fear must be redirected. You are not expected to not feel fear. It's natural and normal, yet you do have the power to make things work in your favor. You can use the power of internal language, creativity, breath and imagination to shift your experience.

Fear is a very important energy to address in this getting healthy journey, because so often you have had your food binges because of a stressful or fearful state. Staying comfortable in that old sequence will keep you stagnant, continually receiving more of the same from your life. More of the same doesn't help you in getting healthy, does it? There has got to be a *shift*.

One day while I was folding and putting away clothes with the television on, Drew Barrymore's E! Entertainment interview about her life caught my attention. In the interview, she was asked how she chooses acting projects. She divulged that if a script she's reading really scares her, she knows she should take the part—when she wonders how the heck she could ever pull it off, and be believable as the character. She knows that just by doing it she'll grow from the experience. That philosophy has stayed with me, and not only do I think about it often, I encourage my Mind Body F.I.T. Club women to do the same.

FEEL FEAR, YET GO FOR IT ANYWAY

It's okay to do things scared. Just be courageous about it! By taking action that is a bit frightening, you will push out the walls of your comfort zone, causing you to grow. Good! You'll develop personally because of it. You may have heard the quote, "Courage is not the absence of fear. It is acknowledging the fear but doing it anyway." I love that beautiful concept. It's fairly simple isn't it? It just requires courage. Remember earlier in the book when I shared with you, courage is the bridge to all high vibration emotions? It's true. Love, freedom, peace, happiness, joy ... they are all reached by way of courage.

Courage is the connector. In order to develop a new way of living in a joyful mind—free of the obsessiveness of food or your weight or the opposite, not caring at all—you'll need courage to stand up to what is no longer working for you. I encourage you to develop a keen sense of awareness in your mind and body. Notice when your energy changes and you get triggered by something. Instead of turning to a food binge, a social media binge or a nasty internal dialogue, practice tuning in. Use the F.I.T. Method to shift the energy. Place your hand on your heart, fixate your eyes as a pattern interrupt and breathe. I invite you to really delve deeper into your body and learn to take command of the sensations within. Know that your mind is always in charge.

The GO Moment

There is a moment that you must recognize in this process of being courageous. It happens when something scares you and your first response is to stop. But now I want you to do the opposite. I call it ... The GO moment. It is an acronym for Growth Opportunity. When you blast open your comfort zone and feel terrified, there is a Growth Opportunity awaiting. Guaranteed. The GO moment happens in the gap between making the decision to move forward despite fear and reaching the other side. It's that space between where you may say, "Oh shit, what have I done?" Living your life in a perpetual state of pushing out of your comfort zone will bring you great rewards. Yes! It is what grows and strengthens your confidence.

WENDY'S STORY

Nine of the Mind Body F.I.T. Club ladies signed up for the infamous Warrior Dash in Southern California. It was a three-mile dirt course with twelve challenging obstacles including mud pits, vertical walls, and 40-foot rope climbs. I wanted my ladies to have an experience that would force them to face their fears. So, we all signed up!

A few months prior, while on a business trip presenting Hypnosis to the U.S. Marine Corps in Japan, I was introduced to the word Bushido. It translates as 'Way of the Warrior'. I thought it would be fun for us to participate in the Warrior Dash as the Bushido Betties, roughly translated as ... Way of the Warrior Woman.

We tied Japanese warrior headbands around our ponytail heads that donned the sign of the red sun, and the symbol for 'Divine Wind'. Our plan was to be courageous. We wore cute custom tees that displayed our warrior name and we banded together like a sixth grade dance troop. At the start line we agreed that our race strategy would be to stay together, help each other through the obstacles and finish as a team. There were some ladies faster than others, but it didn't matter, we knew we were there to have each other's backs.

Wendy, one of the Bushido Betties, had been in my MBFC community for a good amount of time, and had been working hard to create new habits by walking at work during lunchtime, and making better eating choices. She was really beginning to absorb the spirit of our inspiration in the club. Her family could not believe she was doing the Warrior Dash with us. She had never done anything like it in her life. This race was way out of Wendy's comfort zone. Prior to the race, Wendy showed her kids the videos and pictures on the Warrior Dash website, and they called her a hero for having the guts to go do it. She wasn't even sure that she really did have the guts, but she was certainly going to try.

On that day, Wendy had her bouts with disbelief during the first mile. Red in the face and breathing hard, she felt unsure of herself before we even hit the first obstacle. The physical response is an example of the self-perpetuating fear I described above. As a group, we knew Wendy was fighting off self-doubt, so we banded together to cheer her on. At the vertical wall, she was forced to focus in order to make it to the top. That was great! But, then she panicked once she was up there. She felt like she was going to fall. She held on so tightly that she resembled a terrified cat on a rope. We gave her encouragement by shouting, "You got this, Wendy!" I did some quick hypnosis with her on the top to manage the panic attack and get it in control. There's the evidence of the power of mind-body communication. She was able to overcome that moment and smile while up there and we have a picture to prove it!

As we jogged away from the wall, we looked back to sneak a last glance at its menacing presence. Wendy was stunned that she had conquered it. Under the barbed wire and over the 40-foot rope climb, Wendy faced her fears at every obstacle. She was participating in an event that she never even considered would be something she could do. But with the encouragement of like-minded friends and the desire to conquer her body issues (which are actually mind issues), Wendy flailed herself from her comfort zone and grew a new confidence that she will continue to take with her on her journey. She said the entire week after the race felt surreal. She was still grasping to understand how she could be so courageous. She proved to herself that day that she is worth the effort and CAN DO IT. She said on our coaching call the following week that she now truly believes she can do anything she sets her mind to.

Warrior Dash provided Wendy with a beacon of light, revealing to her the path of her journey. Had she not felt the fear and did it anyway, Wendy would not have the gift of belief in herself.

BEWARE, THE SISTER OF
FEAR IS WORRY

Fear and worry go hand in hand synergistically. Had Wendy worried that she would not finish, she may not have even shown up that day. Engaging in worry is using your mind for negative energy. By doing so, you are creating affirmations that are not positive seeds of thought. Are you worried, and making up potential outcomes before you even get started? You may be making up reasons that are not valid; composed of "What ifs?"

What if I can't do it?

I can't run. What if I have a heart attack?

I don't go to the gym. What if I look like the fat girl on the treadmill?

What if this program doesn't work for me?

What if I gain all the weight back?

I'm afraid to walk by myself. What if I get mugged or there are animals loose?

I'm too fat to exercise. What if I hurt myself?

Before you proceed with any more what ifs, fears or excuses, allow yourself the freedom to evolve your thinking. Decide to abandon the old comfort thinking, and attract the people and tools you need, to be successful by directing your mind towards your goals. Better yet, make those goals present in the here and now!

GUIDANCE AND CLAIMING A NEW IDENTITY

I believe that people come into our lives for a specific purpose. It could be that there is a lesson for us to learn, and that person is there to teach it to us. Some are in our lives for a lifetime, others for brief months or a few years. These people are *mentors*. They don't look a certain way or wear a uniform for recognition. They come in many forms and in all walks of life. But they are very useful and vital to our growth.

Our need for human bonding is what enables these soulful connections to create personal growth within us. Knowing that another person believes in you, or sees in you a spark that others don't, is what keeps our hope alive. When another person gets you, it allows you to feel validated and significant in the world. I believe having a mentor is a key component to your personal success.

At one point in my career, while in search of the next level of my growth, I knew that a mentor would be necessary for me to continue an upwardly mobile pace. Many of the personal development leaders that I would listen to spoke about the importance of having mentors in your life. They talked about aligning yourself with people you want to be like and becoming highly selective of your friends; choosing to spend time with those who add value to your life and make you want to strive to be a better person.

At that time, I didn't really have any successful friends. Most of my friends were treading water just like me. And

I don't mean to say that my friends weren't great people. I'm just stating that in my view I knew no one who seemed to have the whole package. Some had money but were really screwed up in their personal lives. Some were very happy people but were totally broke. Others were really good at their career, but they could not seem to keep a relationship together, and others couldn't manage their weight. I wanted the kind of mentor that the leaders had talked about, so I started asking God for a mentor. Or, you could say, I put it out there.

During that time, we had planned a family vacation with my favorite sister-in-law to go to Hawaii. She would bring her two girls, we'd bring our kids, and we'd spend the week soaking up the island vibe. My sister-in-law had started running a couple of years prior and by this time was diligently running four or five times a week. She's a beautiful woman, my same age, with a very outgoing personality and successful in her own right. She had been through an unsettling divorce and a very trying time in her life but had come through it with what I viewed as strength and courage.

I knew my sister-in-law would be bringing her running shoes to Hawaii, and I wanted to keep up with her. After all, she was a woman who I admired. She had qualities that I respected, and those qualities made me want to dig deep and find them within myself. So if she asked me to run with her, then I was prepared to step up to the plate and say, "Yes!"

The day before my plane departed, I went down to my local discount shoe store and purchased a pair of $40 running shoes. I packed them in my carry-on bag and was ready to put them to good use. There is something very important to this story, that you must know—I was not a runner. I had not put on a pair of running shoes since the fifth grade. I was the girl that failed P.E. in high school, because I refused to dress out. I thought polyester was an insult to the fashion industry, so I refused to wear those lame uniforms. Ha! I was more into ditching P.E. and smoking cloves behind the bleachers with the rebellious kids.

Our first morning in Hawaii, I awakened to the sound of the ocean. I could smell the sweet scent of plumeria growing outside our condo window, and I couldn't wait to get out into the island sun.

Just as I predicted, my sister-in-law soon knocked on my condo door. When I opened the door to her cheerful face (she's a morning person) she said, "You wanna go for a jog?" I was pleased to oblige. I looked to her as a woman of confidence, a chick who had direction in her life. I wanted to be around her because of that, so I was excited to engage in an activity with her.

Each morning we jogged down Alii Drive, a palm tree lined road that hugs the white, sandy beaches of the Kona Coast. We'd run 2.5 miles south to a gorgeous public beach, quickly grab a cool drink of water from the faucet and continue the jog back the 2.5 miles to our condos. There were moments I didn't think I could continue, and by day three I had a blister or two on my toes, and my calves were aching. I would crawl out of bed walking like Donald Duck with sore, tight muscles. But, I would stretch, drink some fresh mango guava juice, and I was up for the challenge again.

Our families had an awesome vacation together. The day we left the quaint Kona Village, we all felt relaxed, rejuvenated and happy about the time we had spent together. I got on that Hawaiian flower-clad plane feeling proud of myself. I had run 35 miles that week! I didn't even know I could do that! Had it not been for my superhero sister-in-law, I would not have had that experience, nor the gift of accomplishment. I wouldn't have done it on my own.

A mentor can help you to the next level of your life. They may not even know they are mentoring you, but the point is—when someone shows up in your life who challenges you to be better, be ready to say, "Yes, I'll take that challenge." I had asked for a mentor, and not only did she show up, but she did so with a success tool in hand, in the form of running. Like a relay race, my sister-in-law passed the baton, and enabled me to continue my journey of personal development.

You've already read the many running stories infused throughout this book, so now you know how I became a runner. It was because of my sister-in-law's influence, and not until the age of forty. Continuing the five-mile increments I had run in Hawaii had been a challenge in the hilly terrain of my hometown, but I slowly increased my ability. With continued practice and training, I was able to break through my limitations and run my very first event, a local 10K (6.2 miles). It felt like an incredible accomplishment. At the finish line on that day, I finally claimed I was an actual runner. All the training before that, I denied myself that label. I was an imposter, posing as a runner.

Your identity may be holding you back. Have you ever considered that? Your mind is so powerful, it creates prisons.

Oh that's not me, I don't do that.

I can't start that at this age.

I just fiddle around with it,
I'm not really a _____.

Prove you want it by believing in yourself.

Ask, *Am I willing to face my fears to achieve the healthy lifestyle I want?*

MANTRA
"I observe the fear, but I move forward anyway."

F.I.T. EXERCISE

Do it Scared and With Courage

You are now establishing awareness in recognizing opportunities to grow. Describe a fitness-related experience that scared you but now recognize it as a GO moment (Growth Opportunity).

- Place your hand on your heart for calibration.

- Fixate your eyes.

- Deep breathing.

- Connect with the F.I.T. question.

- With pencil and paper in front of you, journal your answer. Ask your inner thoughts to flow from your mind and onto the paper providing you valuable insight.

What have you learned by facing your fears and in what ways can you borrow that courage and apply it now to your kickass health goals?

_____

_____

_____

_____

_____

_____

_____

What do you now value more than anything, because of
what you've pushed yourself to do?

_____

_____

_____

_____

_____

_____

Who are you becoming? I am becoming ...

_____

_____

_____

_____

_____

_____

_____

I am always pushing the ladies in my programs to expand their comfort zones. I want them to shift how they view themselves. So, when the idea of all of us meeting up to run a half marathon was brought up on the weekly coaching call by our member Trish Kelly, I knew I needed to take my own advice and say, "Yes!"

During that week I went online to check out the details of the race. Thirteen miles was longer than I could imagine. I was nervous about signing up. You've felt that feeling. When you want to do something, but the rush of self-doubt makes you start overthinking it. That little voice inside my head, you know the one; the voice that sometimes says nice things, and other times is mean and sabotaging? That voice kept urging, *Do the full marathon — 26.2 miles. I thought, my gosh, there is no way! I'm no athlete.*

Well, because I truly believe in what I am teaching, and I refuse to listen to limiting self-talk, I decided to listen to my intuition and sign-up for the full, 26-mile marathon. I can remember my hand shaking as I maneuvered my mouse down the sign up page to click on the marathon button. I filled in my information, entered my credit card and clicked Submit. YIKES! I could hardly believe what I just signed up for. I was terrified! I was definitely outside, WAY OUTSIDE, my comfort zone.

Slowly I learned to run longer miles. I subscribed to *Runner's World Magazine* and signed up for an online training program by renowned running coach Hal Higdon. When you commit to something bigger, you start looking for the ways and means to accomplish it. I knew that I needed to learn how one trains to run a marathon. How many miles do I train? How often? What do I eat to fuel my body? What about recovery after runs? I had many questions and searched for resources to answer them.

I steadily increased my strength and stamina. I found it to be liberating and fun. There was a time that I could not fathom running past three miles, but I knew that I had my MBFC ladies counting on me to follow through. I reported in to them on our weekly coaching calls so that we could track each others' progress. My motivation was absolutely to prove it could be done. After all, I was no athlete; just a mother of three with ambition.

Building up to marathon day, I signed up for the City of Angels Half Marathon. The race went from Griffith Park to downtown Los Angeles. I secured reservations at a hotel for the night before the race, and arranged for Mom to accompany me and watch my kids at the hotel. As we drove to Los Angeles, Mom sarcastically made a negative remark about why anyone would want to put themselves through such a terrible experience. "Why would anyone want to run 13 miles?" she said. As usual, Mom was her pessimistic, critical self. Where was the support? The ... *Hey you're going to do great! Gosh, I'm so proud of you for doing something like this.* I chose to not take her words in and get triggered by them. I was growing, and not going to let her own limiting beliefs stop me.

I awoke the next morning at 5:30 a.m. with jitters; nervous about the race. Downing a protein/carb bar, and throwing on my running gear, I headed for the bus pickup that shuttles runners to the start line. I was greeted by a major letdown. Unfortunately, I missed the shuttle, and arrived fifteen minutes after the last scheduled departure. Certainly this was no one's fault but my own. I thought I had all the details in order, but I missed this one SUPER important detail! I thought to myself in sarcastic disgust, *Hello De'Anna there was a time schedule??!!*

I was forced to make a decision; either turn back and not participate, or figure out a way to get to the start line ten miles away. Just then, two women walked up ranting about how they missed the bus too. They said they were going to catch a taxi, and I asked if I could come along with them. I had no money on me, just my cell phone. I was very pleased when they obliged my friendly request. BTW ... always have money, cell phone and ID with you.

The taxi driver took us up and over a Los Angeles hill and continued six or seven miles until we arrived at the closest point to the start line. He pulled over at the intersection, and it was clear the race was just down the way. Race barriers were set up, and policeman stood along the intersection directing traffic. I jumped out of the taxi thanking the two kind women and ran towards what I believed to be the start line. As I hurried, I confirmed with the policemen the direction to the start, and he pointed me down the paved, tree-lined drive.

Jogging down the road, I expected to see the thousands of runners, the volunteers and the big start line excitement any minute. But no such luck. I continued my jogging pace down the road thinking the start line had to be just around the corner when I began to see runners coming toward me going the opposite direction. I realized, *Uh-oh, the race has started! And I'm not in it. Run faster!*

On that sunny December morning, I ran three miles just to get to the start line. My hard-earned months of training lead me to this day to run the 13.1 miles I trained for. But now I was finding myself mentally challenged with the prospect ahead of me that I would be running a 16.1 mile race. Feeling a slight sense of defeat, I jogged on with all the courage I could muster. I did not want to be a quitter. I knew that I must restrategize my thinking, mentally adjust to the idea of running 16.1 miles and basically suck it up.

When I finally arrived at the start line, everyone but one man was gone. The volunteers had already left for the finish line, the tables and easy-up tents were broken down, and the runners were long gone down the road and out of sight. The one race official present was breaking down the trussing at the start line. He saw me running over, and I anxiously asked him, "Am I too late?" He answered, "No, just cross the line so that your electronic tag registers that you are in the race." I did just that, and he pulled the electronic cable up right after I passed.

I was literally the LAST runner in the race. A few yards past the start line, the race official came running up to inform me that I was the LAST runner in the race. This was not something I needed to be informed about, I thought with sarcasm. It was obvious by the abandoned scene. He told me to not feel pressured and to just have fun. I thought, *Yeah, okay, no pressure, there's just 6,210 people ahead of me.* I had not come to win the race, but heck, that was intimidating.

After he left me, I felt a few tears stream down my cheek. My tears were that of celebration and joy, after all, I had to run just to get to the start line. I proved to myself that I wanted to be there. I was committing to complete this race no matter what, and that gave me inspiration under my feet. To enhance my positivity, I decided to count heads. It took me about a mile before I caught up to the last group of runners. Each person that I passed; I would feel good about the fact that I was no longer last. I lost count at one hundred and kept going.

Because I had not trained to run 16.1 miles, the race was a major challenge for me. I started off strong, but by mile 10, which was 13 for me, I wanted to just lay down and sprawl out under a tree. My legs felt like they were no longer part of my body. They were as heavy as tree stumps. I was depleted of energy, and unsure of my fate in finishing the race. The only thing I had to keep me going was my MIND.

Have you ever felt so defeated that you just wanted to crawl under a tree? Or stay in bed? Or not show up to your life? Although I was physically exhausted, I knew I had to get myself down that road to the finish line. My mental strength is what kept me in the race that day. It was PURE DETERMINATION. As the end of the race grew nearer, the sidewalks became more populated with onlookers and family members cheering on their favorite runner. Their energy helped me push my body to a victorious finish; unintentionally running 16.1 miles, and a story and medal to prove it. Even though it had not gone as planned, it was a great day. Running had taught me something very powerful about myself, and for that, I would never take back the unexpected course of events. I learned about motivation that comes from within; the kind of self-reliance that is only learned through doing something challenging. Although every muscle, ligament and tendon in my body ached, I received a gift for my soul.

There were many opportunities during my race day experience when I could have given up. When I missed the bus, I could have gone back to the hotel angry and blamed my mishap on the race coordinators. When I learned the race had already started, I could have disappointingly quit and turned back. When I arrived at the start line and realized I was dead last, I could have said, "Screw It!" But, instead of creating drama and holding myself back, I took personal responsibility and created an opportunity for learning so that I could keep my mobility moving in the right direction. Whoa, who was this woman?! She was the new me.

You've got to reassess your race. Realize the obstacles that have come into your life are not dealbreakers. Reevaluate your plan and expand your comfort zone. Stop asking, *What if?* and start taking action. It will take guts on your part. When a neighbor brings you a plate of cookies as a nice gesture, you have a choice; eat the plate of cookies yourself or eat one and give the rest away. When you've had a stressful day, and your first response is to eat, stop by a grocery store and buy a cake, have the strength to know that devouring it is not part of your new mindset plan. It's really not about the food at all. Because those yummy things can be in your life. You just deserve to believe in yourself versus believing the food will save the day. You are the real hero here.

F.I.T. EXERCISE

Take a Power Pause and Answer
This Soulful Question

- Place your hand on your heart for calibration.

- Fixate your eyes.

- Deep breathing.

INSERT F.I.T. QUESTION

In what ways has your current identity held you back?

_____

_____

_____

_____

_____

What can you take on to expand your self belief and grow your identity?

_____

_____

_____

_____

_____

Chapter 10

Vital Mind Cycles

When your habits and personal identity align with your values, you are assured a healthy mind and a fulfilled life.

~ De'Anna Nunez

I n this chapter I want to expose key insights I've garnered from hundreds of private hypnosis sessions. By doing this amazing work, I've been fortunate to observe psychological patterns that emerge for each person. They exist because the brain and body are so incredible at keeping us safe. But that also means you may be staying too safe in patterns that don't support where you're headed. My goal is to attempt to simplify how these mind cycles operate so you can become more conscious of the unconscious decisions you are making daily.

Inside my examples, I want you to turn yourself inside out for the goal of complete clarity. When you don't have clarity, you can feel unsure, foggy or stuck in your current habits or beliefs. Your mind will tell you things like, "I'm just not that motivated" or "maybe I don't have what it takes." Those thoughts are not truths, they are just the little lies we tell ourselves based on our failed past attempts.

Here's what I so brilliantly observed; the mind cycles exist without question. You just may not be aware of them or know how to change them. They were elusive. Until now. In the next few pages we will design a vital mind cycle that serves as the structure to the new you. Next time you get sidetracked with stink'n think'n or analysis paralysis, or fall into bad habits traps, you'll have a plan.

You'll be savvy on how to shift your unconscious mind cycle back into its most vital.

THERE ARE 5 KEY STAGES TO AN UNCONSCIOUS MIND CYCLE

Consider all that you have experienced; your history, people, places and things that have occurred in your life. The massive amounts of information stored in your subconscious include the joyous and special moments, as well as all the misinterpreted childhood perspectives from traumas, divorce, death, abuse, poverty, love withheld, family order, abandonment and more. In essence, both positive or negative, they are all forms of power that shape your unconscious mind.

These influences cause unconscious beliefs and perspectives that can steal your peace of mind and undermine the goals you are trying to create today. They've shaped who you are, even the habits you have now, have been created from an **unconscious need** based on these influences in your mind. The imprints of those impressionable experiences have created **unconscious cycles** and they form an overall MINDSET. Have you experienced this? You may be on track towards your goal, feeling focused, but then get derailed. What happened?

You got triggered. I know you have experienced it. I sure have! Getting triggered is no fun and it often sends you down the rabbit hole. This is when people like you and me have turned to food to cope. Until now. Listen up. When you get triggered, it's because you have an unconscious need that is not getting met. You do well for a few days or weeks. But when you get triggered, because we all do, the unresolved need is so strong that it interrupts your focus and derails you time and time again, thus reinforcing the cycle. The key to breaking the cycle and forming a new more beneficial one, is making the unconscious conscious. I want you to slow everything down and sharpen your awareness muscles, so that now you see and feel the cycle as it is happening in real time.

THE CORE OF THE CYCLE

Stage 1 – The Need

The cycle is perpetuated by your unconscious programming. It is an unconscious need that requires attention and it's so powerful that it will bark for recognition. For example, a need to "feel good enough." You may have received criticism in your upbringing that left you feeling like you'll never be enough. You've worked your ass off to banish that feeling, fighting for your light. You know undoubtedly your light and brilliance is in there. But the "not good enough" feeling is like a shadow that follows you. You keep trying to outrun it or juke it.

Stage 2 – The Trigger (or Cue)

Some days you're brave enough to stop and go toe to toe with it, staring it down. Other days, you curl up in the fetal position while it screams at you. This is what it feels like to get *triggered* by an unconscious need. Stage 2 happens when emotions flair from work stress, family stress, fears, loneliness, etc., and your unconscious need says, *You are never enough.*

Stage 3 – The Habit

To avoid feeling those heartachingly uncomfortable emotions, your mind creates diversions in the form of unconscious *habits*. It's as if you go into a trance state and do what you do to fulfill the need. This is when you eat when you're not even hungry. Stage 3 is when the habit temporarily soothes or quiets the unconscious need.

Stage 4 – Temporarily Satisfied

Once you've completed the habit stage, you're in stage 4, and you now feel *temporarily satisfied*. Your need has been tempered with pleasure for the time being. Yet, here's the tragedy. Your real need, the need to feel good enough, has still not been addressed or resolved.

Stage 5 – Credit the Habit

You credit your *habit routine* for comforting you, thus reinforcing your dependence on the habit. You're convinced food is your friend and you can't imagine living your life without its companionship.

Stage 6 – The Belief

The *unconscious belief* is powerfully reinforced that you will never get your needs met. This stage is where you make up all kinds of stories and beliefs about who you are and what you are missing in your life. Until you resolve and release the NEED vying for attention underneath the surface, you will always seek temporary pleasure and get derailed. It's an endless loop that causes you more pain and an unstable mindset.

This entire cycle is unique to everyone. For some, the cycle may be based on a core belief that feels positive. Many people enjoy the habit of eating because their unconscious core need is a feeling of love-connection from family. Perhaps your unconscious patterns are connected to food as a celebration, treat, family time, special moments. Therefore, when you get triggered by the stresses of life, the first thing you want to do is retreat to the safety and security of that unconscious feeling. The habit of turning to food to fulfill that need is triggered, and the cycle begins.

When you have a goal to be at your healthiest body weight, but the habit of food intake is in place to fulfill your needs, you'll have trouble ever sustaining your weight easily. Your belief as exampled in stage 6 will become the untrue truth that food is part of your culture, or, it's just how you need to operate. Recognize that these habit routines can be many things such as over-spending, smoking, sex, drinking, etc. Deep-seated habits are only in place to mask a need. Uncover the need, and you are well on your way to release from the negative cycle that has felt so gripping.

Don't be dismayed. Truth is, you have 100% power over all of it. You can reveal, release and recode. Your struggle or *unconscious need* is also your greatest teacher. It keeps popping up for a reason. It wants and deserves attention. I urge you to *work with it.*

You keep trying to overcome your internal needs by overcompensating, proving yourself or avoiding it altogether. But instead, I'm suggesting that you use it as a cue to heal yourself and become the best version of you.

You get to have your needs met and become fulfilled. The very thing you want to have in your life, you can. The very thing you want to be, you can be. You want to feel and be good enough? Acknowledge it now. You want to feel love and joy? Acknowledge that now. Total acceptance.

3 STEPS THAT WILL CAUSE YOUR NEXT BREAKTHROUGH

Are you ready to fertilize your needs and allow your healthy mindset cycles to flourish? Let's go.

— Step 1 —

Release from the need to blame, avoid or be stuck in a loop of wanting. Take responsibility for your *self management* and happiness. Make the unconscious conscious, and increase the awareness of what needs you have and how they can be consciously fulfilled, nourished and celebrated in new ways.

— Step 2 —

View this new self-awareness as a gift, and design habits and beliefs that actually fulfill your needs.

— Step 3 —

Change your perspective about the unconscious need. *See your struggle as the very gem that has shaped your core values today.*

I'm willing to be extra vulnerable and share with you a few ways this all unfolded for me and truly liberated me.

FOOD, SEX AND MONEY

Now that's a great heading. If that doesn't get your attention? Ha!

Example 1: Breakthrough

Mom and I always struggled in our relationship. Instead of holding resentment, I use that experience as an anchor to knowing it's one of my core values. I value communicating with my children and loving them unconditionally. It's what I get to do. I thank Mom for unknowingly showing me that.

Core Value – I used to use food to fill the void of feeling unloved. Now I am meeting my own needs by reaching out to my kids, husband and friends with love, recognizing that I truly value connection and appreciate strong relationships above all else. I can now manage a healthy weight more effortlessly because I don't turn to food to self-soothe.

Example 2: Breakthrough

Growing up, my parents fought about money relentlessly. It took them seven years to get divorced due to fighting about assets. That was my environment growing up. I found myself as an adult chained down by money struggles. I would make it and spend it, not feel good enough to charge what I was really worth for my services and at times put myself in unsafe and unstable situations with a lack of mindset.

Core Value – As I took a deeper look within myself, I uncovered all the untrue truths I was holding around money. I recognized where the beliefs came from and forgave all parties involved. Deepening my emotional intelligence around money allowed me to take responsibility and develop new habits and beliefs. I went from deflecting money to attracting money, and now have confidence in myself I never thought I would have.

Example 3: Breakthrough

As a young girl I experienced multiple male teachers who gave me extra attention. Dad was not around as I wanted or needed. Not because he didn't want to be, but because Mom was bitter and discouraged his participation. I was a girl with *Daddy issues*. The attention from these male teachers made me feel smart and beautiful. In reflection, these teacher relationships were very odd and inappropriate, but at the time they filled a void. I learned to bat my eyes and charm them with my outgoing personality. They played the game just as I did. The need for male attention was a strong unconscious need. As a result, I became promiscuous and used beauty and charm in ways that attracted what I thought I needed but almost always left me feeling used and depleted. The habit never truly fulfilled the need. It also caused me to brutally beat myself up with mean internal language and feelings of worthlessness. Breaking through this unconscious need was one of my biggest shifts ever because it was also so intricately intertwined with my body, the need to diet and look good and the despair I felt when I was unattractively overweight (or so I thought).

Core Value – Healing this need became a gift of understanding a true sense of sexuality, self-love and self-worth. Exercise and eating well is not attached to any dysfunctional unmet needs. Exercise and eating well is all for me and is a pure source of self-care.

I share these very private examples because it is my deepest desire to be brave with my emotions and a warrior with my soul's purpose. My life's work is meant to be your bridge. For you to see yourself in a new light and let go of the shackles of the past, is the most amazing thing you can ever do for yourself and those in your circles. Not only will your life change, but the lives of those who encounter your bravery and brilliance will also change.

COMMIT TO MASTERY

The secret of success is learning how to use pain and pleasure instead of having pain and pleasure use you. If you do that, you're in control of your life. If you don't, life controls you.

~ Tony Robbins

Discovering your unconscious need is vital to developing a deeper understanding of yourself. Shifting the need into your core values will provide you a foundation for amazing self-care.

A Vital Mind Cycle is You ...

- Getting your unconscious needs met in a healthy manner

- Managing your mindset daily

- Leveraging your core values for reinforcement

- Getting involved in your success

By practicing this process as a way of life, you are choosing happiness and true fulfillment. Let's take a look at how shifting the cycle changes everything. Below is the same woman with the same issue, but she's doing something about it.

A Vital Mind Cycle Based on the Former Example

Stage 1 – The Need

She needs to feel like she's enough, therefore she takes responsibility for fulfilling that need in healthy ways.

Stage 2 – The Trigger

She gets triggered by work stress, family stress, etc. but recognizes that she can think of it as a cue or reminder to stay in a healthy pattern. She knows to breathe, manage her mind and recognize what's really going on.

Stage 3 – The Routine or Habit

She puts on her walking shoes and goes out the door later that day. Her mind shifts while she's out there and she begins to feel proud of herself for taking control. She sorts though her struggle, listens to her self-talk with a compassionate ear, and makes necessary adjustments in her mindset. Rather than blaming herself for not being good enough, she solves the actual problem with a more objective response.

Stage 4 – Satisfaction

She feels fulfilled, recognizing that exercise is a form of self-love and self-management. She takes responsibility for her own healthy practices and tells herself, "Good job."

Stage 5 – The Credit

She credits herself for making the effort and stays in the flow of a growth mindset.

Stage 6 – The Belief

Her belief and mindset is that healthy practices are an integral part of her happiness. She does not depend on an outside source to give it to her. She feels a sense of power, confidence and personal responsibility. Her needs have been met in a healthy manner. She is fulfilled and knows how to repeat the cycle and stay in a strong mindset.

TEST YOUR THEORIES AS A SCIENTIST

The key to successfully managing your mindset and overcoming your own pitfalls is to take on the role of the scientist. Learn to be an explorer of your own truths and investigate your habits and beliefs with an air of non-judgement. Connect the dots back to the original source where the mindset or belief was adopted by the subconscious. In doing so you are treating the source, not the symptom. Root cause versus outcome.

Ask yourself the following questions.

F.I.T. EXERCISE

Close your eyes, take 5 deep inhales and exhales. Answer the questions with your emotions, not your analytical thoughts. This is so important! Let your emotions guide the way. Go with gut feeling, not 'thinking hard'.

Exploration Questions to Help You Flesh Out Your Mindset Cycle

What is one habit that seems to derail you, and you want to change?

_____

_____

_____

We only do something if we believe it serves us on some level. So overlook the obvious and dig deep into your emotional needs. This is your unconscious need that is not being met.

Where, when or from whom did you learn the behavior or belief? Truth is, you didn't always do it. It started from something. What is that something? Follow the timeline of your life back to the cause and journal about it here:

_____

_____

_____

What do you think you get out of it by continuing the behavior?

_____

_____

As you let go of blaming the original source, and take full responsibility for developing a Vital Mindset, what action can you take to still get your needs met, yet do it more healthfully and to your real benefit that aligns with core values and purpose?

_____

_____

_____

Decide how you can leverage the cycle to work in your favor.

You can:

- Get your needs met.
- Do it in a healthy way rather than suffering or causing yourself harm or unwanted habits.
- Be honest with the 'need' you are really trying to fulfill.
- Align your mindset cycle with core values and purpose.

My core values are:

_____

_____

_____

Identify and Shift into a Vital Mind Cycle:

_____

_____

_____

Negative Mindset Cycle: *(the old you)*

"I need_____. I get triggered by_____
so I _____and then I feel temporarily satisfied. I
believe I need it in my life for survival and sanity."

Vital Mindset Cycle: *(the new you)*

"I need_____. I get triggered by_____ so
I _____and feel fulfilled and successful. I believe
in my greater purpose, feel peace of mind and love life."

Never stop practicing **The Art of Your Healthy Mindset
Cycle.**

When you transition from, *"I'm not where I want to
be because ..."* to *"I see the lessons in my struggle and
how they've shaped my core values. I now know what's
important to me and I'm grateful for my struggle as I also
see it as my strength. I am honored to do this work and
practice as a master would."*

Dig deep within for strength and discipline.
You're worth it, and you're not in it alone.

~ De'Anna Nunez

ONE AMAZING HABIT

To accomplish something big, a thing you've never done
before, you'll be required to grow into it. You'll need to
take the same you, and innovate yourself. Innovation
essentially means to do something differently so the
same thing looks and feels entirely new.

This is the part where you're going to see how this big thing, like maintaining your healthiest body for good, can actually happen. Yes! You've laid the foundation by getting super clear with understanding yourself better. Now it's time to put the vision into motion and take action. But how? You might be thinking, *I've had dreams and visions and goals before and I didn't follow through. What makes this different?*

A large part of success is believing that you can have it and granting yourself permission. Successful people have success-habits. Therefore, belief and habits are components of the same strong root or cycle. Are you ready to make your success easier? I will teach you how to set yourself up to win by breaking your actions down into bite-sized pieces you know you can accomplish.

In running marathons, I learned to simplify long distances into phases that I knew I could accomplish. Otherwise, the big was too big for my mind. I would often feel a barrage of self-doubt when I focused on the big, so instead I found a way to make it believable. You may experience that too when you think of the amount of weight you want to lose, or the commitment it might take.

You have a vision of what you want to look like, be like, feel like, and to accomplish that it's vital that you focus on what you can control right now. Today. We are innovating a process to make it easier for you to succeed. It's all mindset. Do you want to stay the same, or are you ready to change? Innovation requires an experimental mindset.

The Golden Rule of Habit Change: You can't extinguish a bad habit, you can only change it.

~ Charles Duhigg, PhD. Behavior Scientist & Author of the *Power of Habit*

HOW DO YOU MAKE VISION A REALITY?

I'm about to introduce you to the **One Amazing Habit** philosophy. Regular running became my *One Amazing Habit* that matched up with my goal to run a marathon. But then I realized, running (or any consistent exercise) was the glue that held my fitness mindset together. So why would I ever want to stop doing that?

I ask you ...

What *One Amazing Habit* aligns with your goal?

Through a process, we are going to unveil your key *One Amazing Habit*. That way you can give your incredible focus to the right thing that will actually make all the difference.

There is ONE habit that is so aligned with your goal that it becomes the obvious action you must engage in regularly to make progress. Now, not only is it the pathway to the goal, it also causes an emotional stir or fire within you. It's that thing you actually can learn to really enjoy. You've just been pulled in so many directions that you haven't prioritized it or allowed yourself to actually love it. Your goal is not just an achievement of a thing, it's an achievement of who you become because of it. It is all-encompassing, adding layers of depth and meaning to the legacy of your life.

Let's begin.

Identify HOW you'll make your GOAL happen > HABIT is the actionable fuel.

Step 1 Instructions: Write out the key actions that are required for you to achieve your goal below. Make a list below of all the actions that will be required of you.

1 _____

2 _____

3 _____

4 _____

5 _____

6 _____

7 _____

8 _____

9 _____

10 _____

Next, review the above with a keen eye and decide with process of elimination, what is the *One Habit* listed above that causes your other habits to fall into place more automatically?

Ask yourself, which *One Action* is worthy of becoming a habit and has the power to create a natural ripple effect on the others?

There is science behind the *One Amazing Habit*. It's been identified as a keystone habit, which has the ability to do two powerful things.

1. This type of habit is so powerful that it automatically causes other habits to fall in line.

2. A Keystone Habit *(One Amazing Habit)* can actually change your identity (who you believe you are).

For example, when I first started running it was really hard. But I was inspired to keep going because I was leading the Mind Body F.I.T. women and it seemed to be something I could maintain while traveling. I hadn't run since elementary school. It was a brand new learning curve as an adult. You've already read the many running stories within this book so you know how it turns out with me eventually running marathons and ultra marathons. Perhaps you remember the story of running my first 10K where I felt like a total outsider? Although I had been running 3-4 times a week for months, I still felt like I wasn't really a runner. Here's where the analogy of the *One Amazing Habit* kicks in.

That one habit of running regularly caused me to create a

keystone habit. Within it contained the two differentiating factors of what sets this habit apart from all other little minor habits.

Keystone Habit:

When I run in the run morning, I come home feeling confident and ready to conquer my day. I immediately drink water.

Identify your *One Amazing Habit* and write it here big and loud.

_____

_____

_____

_____

_____

_____

_____

_____

In the next chapter, you will learn simple and effective mindset strategies that you can apply to eating. I have shared these insights with women across the nation, and along with all the other insights, it has helped many of them lose one hundred pounds the natural way! You will learn how to direct your mind toward your goals and begin to love the foods that will help you attain the body you want. The best part is, you'll be able to maintain it too. Making an eating choice starts in your mind. And that is precisely where I will help you to make a mindshift in how and what you eat. You may never look at food the same way!

Chapter 11

Mindfull Eating and More

If hunger is not the problem, then
eating is not the solution.

~ Anonymous

Food, glorious food! Just like the song from the age-old play *Oliver* on Broadway, food is glorious and does taste scrumptious. We celebrate with food when we get together with friends and family, parties, holidays and special occasions. That's perfectly acceptable and to be expected. The entire world does that! The goal is not to stop loving food and gathering to break bread with those you love. The goal is to not depend on it for your emotional comfort. The goal is to be free of obsession.

I imagine you've wondered. How did I get here with food? When did I become so dependent or fixated? It's all innocent enough. Our taste buds are vibrantly alive, and when food comes in contact with our taste sensors, it triggers off an emotional response. The taste of food makes us feel good and we want to do it again and again. Blending emotion with food becomes an unconscious formula. We cry with food when suffering a breakup. We feel less lonely when we have food to curl up with on the couch, or to accompany us while on the computer. Food is an easy fix, readily accessible to get our hands on, and it delivers maximum reward. Unlike other drugs, we can use in public and no one notices or cares. In fact, it's encouraged. Yet, the formula of eat and be happy has some major cracks in it, if eating is what you depend on to be happy.

As you've learned throughout this book, your mind and

subconscious can change. The entire process of change will be that much easier and fluid when you let go of the need to tie emotional support to food altogether. Does just the thought of not turning to food trigger an emotional response? What will I do without my favorite nighttime snack? Without my sweet drink? It's my coping mechanism! I promise, you're going to be better for it. My deepest desire is for you to have a peaceful mind and get your real needs met.

YOU CAN ONLY CHANGE A PERSPECTIVE BY BROADENING A PERSPECTIVE

Consider that it's time to create a new perspective on what food can really do for you. ***Food is literal energy for our bodies.*** We cannot survive without nourishment. As our intricate system breaks down the food we ingest, it prepares to send nutrients to many different areas of the body. The body's nourishment process is brilliant, but let's be honest, you may not be eating just to deliver nutrients to your cells, you are often eating because of taste, emotion, habits and subconscious associations. You may have forgotten food's true purpose, and you are utilizing eating time for your purpose—emotional well-being. How often have you chosen your meal selection based on how you feel? Think to yourself for a moment ... do you say, "Hmmm, what do I feel like eating?"

What I'd like to accomplish in this chapter is a mindshift in regard to what you choose to put in your mouth. I'd like to help you begin to recognize food as ENERGY. My goal is for you to be able to look at several food choices, and absolutely know which is the right choice for fat-burning, muscle-fuel and energy. Beyond just knowing, my higher purpose is for you to want to make that choice. It is imperative that you engage in mental reconditioning. I'll help you create the process of shifting your mind. I'll provide you with a new perspective, and F.I.T. Session Exercise Tools to help you solidify your new thinking within the subconscious. With your empowered new thinking, you can then begin the process of putting it into action.

BEGIN TO DECIPHER A
TRICK FROM A TREAT

Homemade hot fudge sundaes don't really satisfy you. Okay, you might have just said, "Bull-oney, De'Anna, hot fudge sundaes are to die for!" Let me explain further. Think about your favorite food for a moment. *The food that you find yourself drawn to even though sometimes you try to regulate how often you eat it.* Now to be healthier, you know you may need to curb your desire for that food, but perhaps the thought of having to let it go makes you feel reluctant. You may be convinced that you cannot live without it.

I would like to suggest that somewhere along your life that particular food gave you the kind of comfort, or emotional fulfillment that you needed. Perhaps your mom served it as a treat, and when you eat it, you feel like you're home. Or, maybe a few chocolates are exactly what you need when feeling stress. Just a few really helps to take the edge off and provides you with relief. That food resonates with you, speaks to your emotions, and it makes you feel good. Think back to the time of your life when you started eating that favorite food. Whatever was going on in your life when you began to rely on food to make you feel better was not about hunger, it was about the emotional state that you were experiencing.

YOU HAVE CREATED A FOOD+EMOTION CONNECTION, AND IT'S POWERFUL

Your emotional connection with food may also be cultural, whereas food is the center of the family. There may be a heavy influence from the region you are from, or traditions that are followed through generations. Heavy sauces, cheeses, pastas, and frying may simply be the way your family has always cooked. These methods have become ingrained in your habits, and traditional cooking evokes a feeling of family. It's a treat that you love indulging in and gives you a feeling of security. In other words, comfort food. That treat you love so much is merely a trick! Your emotions are playing tricks on you through the food that you are sure makes you feel better. It is wearing an *'I love you and will always be here for you'* costume. It's a disguise.

Food is not responsible for your mental and emotional state. There is something really important that I want you to mentally and emotionally grasp. *Remind yourself—you are no longer who you were.* What emotionally fulfills you now may be very different from what fulfilled you then. There may have been circumstances going on that felt out of your control, so you turned to food to help you cope or make you feel better.

Are those same circumstances happening now? Most likely the answer is no. Yet, you are still holding on to a habit that is of the person you were in the past. It's time to let this go! Take the costume off the food that has been disguising itself as love or stress relief and focus on who you want to be. If your challenges are not just in the past, and you are experiencing challenges now, turning to food is not the answer. Food is a temporary coping mechanism. You are in the right place to help you get it all in perspective.

In the Mind Body F.I.T. Program Change Up Your Life Challenge there is a section on emotions and food. It's called *Emotions Pack a Punch!* The materials propose the idea that food is powerful when combined with emotional state. When you eat to satisfy your emotional needs, you will find yourself with a stomach that is never full.

When you say, "Mmmmm that sounds good," know that your connection to your favorite indulgent food is more emotional than you thought. Try it. Close your eyes and have the courage to ask yourself these questions. Ask yourself, does the statement, "Mmmmm that sounds good," reach past your taste buds and into your emotions? Does thinking about eating that food make you feel happy and satisfied before you have even eaten it? If so, you are cluing into a *food+emotion connection.*

If you are one to engage in this food+emotion connection, know that when you eat a food for reasons other than health and nourishment, the rules suddenly begin to change. If you are not on top of your game and don't have your emotional well-being in check, it is a dangerous and vicious cycle that holds on tight. Empower yourself with understanding your food associations.

Through the MBFC subconscious integration tools, Jaylene learned her food associations were established long ago. She considers peanuts to be her ultimate weakness. When she starts eating them, she feels like she just can't stop with a few, it has to be handfuls. She loves them! With careful and compassionate exploration, she discovered her food association was connected to her loving grandparents. In her own home, she was being sexually abused by her father. Yet, she felt safe and comforted in the home of her grandparents and recalls them always having a bowl of peanuts on the coffee table. Her young mind equated peanuts to represent safety and comfort. As an adult, her subconscious followed that formula. Peanuts = safety and comfort. The peanuts can truly never give her the safety and comfort she really valued. Only Jaylene can do that for herself, and she did learn how through her own healing. Like Jaylene, you can move forward without the habits and associations of the past. Rewiring this psychological and emotional connection can be done.

Taking action is key — you must be committed. From this moment forward, you must be fully present while eating your snacks and meals. I am asking you to start eating with your conscious mind, rather than with your emotions, stress or past experiences.

GET IN THE KNOW

Keeping your nutritional intake in check is crucial to your success. It doesn't matter what you eat; if you're eating too many useless calories, you'll gain weight or have trouble maintaining your body's natural ideal weight. If we consume more than we burn, we gain. If we burn more than we consume, we lose. Of further importance, is the quality of each calorie. Even though a cookie and an apple may have the same amount of calories, it's fairly obvious that the apple is a better choice. It provides nutrients, enzymes, and fiber that the cookie does not. Having enough fiber in your daily intake is vital to your body's metabolism. People in general buck this simple concept. Why? Because that means you have to regulate yourself. You have to be mindful of the amount of calories you consume, say no to certain foods, and say yes to others. It's a matter of self-discipline. But, in general, you don't want to have to discipline yourself. You want it to be easy.

It seems easier to just take a pill, not feel hungry, and let the pounds melt off. But a pill won't teach you what you need to know to continue your success. Popular diet centers that provide you with prepackaged foods are just a grocery store with marked up pricing. Their products will give you a visual of the right portion sizes, but they won't teach you about the intricate inner workings of your behaviors. They'll just get you hooked on buying their foods. These are not solutions to the problem, merely Band-Aids. It's temporary.

You must develop personally from the inside out; learn new skills, practice discipline and live with personal integrity. When you say you want to get healthy, stick with it, do what it takes, learn a new normal. This is why the understanding of your mind and behaviors is so crucial. It is absolutely the starting point to your success and the key to continuing that success through weight maintenance for a lifetime.

Living by the basic science of calories in/calories out is fundamental. But in order to truly live by that simple equation, it will take more than just monitoring what food goes in your mouth. Your success will be contingent upon your deeper strength, your commitment to living healthy and your willingness to disconnect from emotional eating.

Don't freak out, there is still room for enjoyment of taste in the scientific equation of calories in/calories out. And, you still get to keep your integrity intact. Once you take out the emotional aspect, food becomes what it is intended to be. Now, because I am a girl that enjoys ice cream, I do like to indulge in my favorite treat on a weekly basis. But, in order to do so, I learned to be mindful. I've gone from eating straight from the half gallon container (back when I was a yo-yo dieter) to a cereal bowl (during my path to healing), all the way down to a 3 oz side serving dish that I don't even need to blink twice about in terms of calorie consumption. And, I don't feel deprived one bit. This is life balance!

I have found a way to *have my cake and eat it too* (except it's ice cream). My secret to developing discipline is utilizing the **GO Moment** tool. Each time I felt a craving, I would ask myself one of two questions, *Am I really hungry? and/or What am I really feeling right now?*

I learned that most of the time, I was eating energy zapping foods to satisfy my emotional needs.

Next time you are digging through the refrigerator, or about to go through the drive thru, ask yourself, *Am I eating for hunger or out of emotion?* If it is because you are hungry, ask yourself the next question, *Will this food I am choosing give me energy, or take my energy away?* In other words, will it be contributing to my fitness or sluggishness? The food on your plate should be as balanced as your emotional well-being. As you begin to create conscious awareness, you'll automatically start eating food for its true intention—for energy!

The Mind Body F.I.T. Club has a tested and proven F.I.T. Meal equation for optimal fat burning.

Lean Protein + Vegetables = Fat Burning

To add necessary macro variety to that equation, add healthy fats, fiber and plenty of hydration.

A one- or two-egg omelet with chopped vegetables is a perfectly balanced starter to your day. Mango chicken and delicious grilled vegetables are a yummy fat-burning lunch. A tablespoon of real almond butter and fresh cut apples makes a mouthwatering snack or desert. And for dinner, try fresh broiled fish with an accompaniment of baked sweet potato fries and steamed broccoli. Rounding out the balance includes good oils/fats, fruits and whole grains. There's also a variety of vegan and vegetarian options with high protein and complex carbohydrates such as edamame, tempeh, nuts, quinoa, chia seed, lentil, tofu, pumpkin seeds and more. Many of these foods, you know to eat. But that doesn't' mean you do it!

Until now.

To become leaner and more fit, eating when you're actually hungry and including the F.I.T. Meal equation when constructing your meals will get you to your goals at a consistent pace.

Conscious Treats

Indulge in a treat and do so with conscious thinking. Doing so will prevent your treat from tricking you into out of control episodes. I recommend scheduling your treats on your calendar. For example, Saturday frozen yogurt at your favorite shop. Scheduling your treats will help you become more conscious when you eat, and it will keep you out of daily mindless overeating.

SANDY'S STORY

My client Sandy came to me to help her lose weight. She's prediabetic and therefore knows to watch her sugar intake. She has cravings for sugar frequently and feels those cravings are her biggest obstacle. As we reviewed her daily eating habits, we revealed two major factors that were making Sandy's health journey feel extra hard. The first one is the actual foods she was consuming regularly. Sandy was buying the 100 calorie pack snacks distributed by her favorite weight loss brand Weight Watchers. They were various types of crackers and she was eating them regularly as her chosen snacks all the while thinking they were a healthy choice.

Now remember, Sandy is concerned about her glucose levels. Yet, what she didn't realize is those snack packs are pure carbohydrates that translate to glucose (sugar) once ingested. A lean protein and veggie is a much better choice to regulate Sandy's metabolism and will also put an end to the constant trap of her body craving excess carbohydrates (sugar). The second factor to making Sandy's healthy improvement easy was to uncover her desire for sweets. I asked Sandy questions that probed her deeper connection to sweets.

I learned about her childhood and that she grew up poor. Her mom made meals that would feed the family but there were never snacks in the house, nor did they grab snacks on the way home from school as a casual outing like many of her friends did. They didn't have extra money to do that. Snacks were reserved for a

Friday night treat as the whole family would go into town and have a soda and a snack. Friday nights were something she looked forward to every week! We revealed that Sandy made a decision way back then. And it was, "When I get older, I'm going to have enough money to treat myself anytime I want to." As an adult, Sandy always kept snacks in the house and feels so happy to give out treats to her grandkids readily.

Sandy had about one hundred pounds to lose, was threatened with looming diabetes and felt desperate to lose the weight. She couldn't figure out why it was so hard to control her cravings and had given up on herself so many times thinking she was destined to be fat. She just didn't have the self-control it must take. Once we revealed her unconscious connection, she was stunned. Sandy had no idea she was sabotaging her own efforts with an outdated, unconscious decision she made sixty-five years ago.

F.I.T. EXERCISE

Food + Emotion

Play a game of connect the dots. Utilize the left column to write down your go-to foods that you eat in high stress situations or as a regular comfort.

Then connect the food with the emotion that is most fitting to the right. It is not necessary to fill up the entire left column. Write in as many foods that you can think of that tend to call your name.

Foods	Emotion
	Fear
	Unlovable
	Loneliness
	Happiness
	Abandoned
	Sadness
	Dejected
	Resentment
	Anger
	Anxiety
	Celebratory
	Frustration
	Stress
	Joy
	Despair
	Guilt
	Grief

YOUR F.I.T. JOURNAL ~ MINDFULL GARDEN

Keeping a **daily food journal** is still the best way to manage your food intake. What can be measured, can be managed. Yes, I know it's old school, but we're going to put a new school twist on it. By food journaling in the way that I suggest, you will expose your poor food choices and reveal the unconscious associations. Practicing awareness is going to put you in a power position with your food intake. Remember, we are shifting you from being out of control, to being gloriously IN CONTROL. You can only do that by getting real with yourself. In order to begin relinquishing your old unconscious eating cycles, you have to get in the know. Studies show that women are 74% more successful at losing weight when they take the time to write down what they are eating. Think of it as empowering yourself! You've heard the saying, "Failing to plan is a plan to fail." I can't agree more. Your food journal is an excellent tool for planning.

I want you to call this very special food journal your Mindfull Garden. We are going to take the old tried and true method of writing food intake down and uplevel it to make it F.I.T. As you focus inward and target your food choices, the Mindfull Garden will assist you in creating new neurological pathways. The concept is to begin associating foods with a metaphor of weeds and flowers. The weeds represent emotional-based choices and/or unbeneficial choices. The flowers represent positive nutritional choices that provide nutritional energy.

The overall goal of your Mindfull Garden is to have a colorful drawing of flowers that represent your many nutritional food choices throughout the day. This process creates subconscious positive associations with food. Each day is an opportunity to discover your strengths and weaknesses, connect with your inner self, and understand your challenges. It's a form of personal therapy that is healing.

It is to be expected that you'll have weeds in your garden. The goal is not to have a weed-free life. Every garden grows weeds just as every human has personal challenges! But the best gardeners stay on top of the weeds by regularly cultivating the garden, getting in there and managing it. Fertilizing and watering it. Imagine if you never weeded or cultivated your garden. It would be overtaken. Have you ever felt overtaken by life's weeds? This metaphor plays to your emotional health and well-being. Are you regularly managing your emotional health and your state of mind? Are you in a continual process of letting go of what no longer serves you? Pulling those weeds and planting new seeds will be you stating your claim to a beautiful, healthy life.

There is a journal resource for you on my website at MindBodyFitLife.com but you can also create your own.

Instructions:

Morning Mindset Focus Prompts:
I value my life, therefore today I am...

(Internal) What can I think or feel to be fulfilled today and maintain a sense of joy?

(External) What can I manage in my environment today, to assure I stay focused on my intentions and best life?

Evening Reflection Prompts:

I am proud of myself for having the courage to...
One Amazing Habit: What I noticed today as a result of prioritizing was...
What I observed about my thinking habits today...
Pull Weeds: Who or what am I choosing to release, let go of or forgive?
My affirmation for sleeping peacefully is...

Your journal should always be close at hand. If you put it away and let it collect dust, you won't get the opportunity to review and experience your progress. Measuring your progress is essential to keep yourself motivated, on track and shed light on your unconscious mind. Perhaps keep it at your bedside to draw in your flowers (and weeds) each day.

THE GOLDEN GROCERY LIST

With a nutrient packed grocery list in hand, shopping will become a well thought out educational experience. At Christmastime, do you write out a list? You most likely write a list of who you want to buy presents for, what presents you're going to buy and how much it's going to cost. Without a list, you may find yourself at the store overwhelmed, confused and spending way more than you had originally planned. Your list keeps you focused, right?

Think of your weekly Golden Grocery List the same way. If you were to go to the grocery store and pull random items off the shelves based on what looks good, you would not only spend more, but you would most likely come home with items that are unhealthy and unfitting to your healthy lifestyle plan. Do not buy the foods that you know sabotage your efforts. If you're having a weak moment in the market, just walk on by. I've had ladies in my Mind Body F.I.T. Club Program go as far as having it out with a food right there in the middle of the market. I'm not kidding, they have actually had a one-sided conversation with their favorite chips. Glaring at the bag saying, "You are not coming home with me. I know what you're trying to do, you're trying to get me to buy you. But no way, I'm not doing it. You're not going to sabotage me."

Be very aware of sneaky marketing. Many food companies like to splash catchy phrases like "Low Fat" "Low Carb" "Gluten Free" "Sugar Free" on their packaging. Or, they strategically place pictures on the label that we associate with health—like pictures of vegetables, a cow or a sun. Don't be fooled. You are a smart, intelligent woman in charge of her health. Would you give up your ability to stay in control by falling for their slick marketing advertising whose job is to make money by selling their food? Your job is to be smart about what you buy and ultimately what you eat.

Getting in the habit of reading nutrition labels is an important step to making the right choices in your meal planning. When I am shopping at the grocery store, there is not a box, can or package that goes unread before it gets dumped into my cart. I want to know what is in the food I am consuming, and if it doesn't pass my test, it goes back.

I have two Golden Agreements:

- No sugar

- No processed fats or fillers

If it has either of these two in the first five ingredients, it goes back. Let's clarify the many names of these culprits, so that you recognize them in an ingredient list.

- Sugar = high fructose corn syrup, brown rice syrup, sugar, organic sugar, honey, fructose, agave syrup, maple syrup, sucrose, glucose, dextrose, evaporated cane juice, maltodextrin, galactose, dextrin, beet sugar, raw sugar, brown sugar, white sugar, concentrated fruit juice, syrup, sorghum

- Fillers = Grains that breakdown as sugar = wheat flour, enriched flour, white flour, cornstarch, tapioca, processed cereals and crackers, cakes, cookies

- Processed fats = hydrogenated vegetable oil, cottonseed oil, lard

If it doesn't state *whole grain*, it is not really wheat. It only has to be 5% wheat to be qualified as wheat bread. That means, the other 95% is processed white flour that has been stripped of its nutrients and fiber. Anything less than *whole grain* (white rice, white bread, wheat crackers, cereal, etc.) is just filler. It's like the dog food industry using cornmeal as its major ingredient. It's just crappy filler. Your body doesn't need that and neither do your dogs. Be sure to choose *whole grain* for your all important complex carbohydrates and never eat them without adding a protein to balance your metabolism.

I'll tell you the God's honest truth, it is frustrating when 70% of what I pull off the shelf is not worthy of my consumption. Yet, I do not cave and buy crappy food because it is easier. Thankfully, we do have markets that are geared towards healthier products; Whole Foods, Trader Joe's, Kowalski's, Jimbo's. Find stores in your area that cater to people who care about their health and nutrition. It may cost a bit more, but it's food that is worthy of your hard-earned dollar. Your body will love you for it. The highly proclaimed documentary *Food, Inc.* says, "Think of purchasing organic foods as your vote to the government demanding a better system for mass food production."

Eating for energy is the method that I have used to maintain my shape. I look at foods with a F.I.T. perspective, and I practice my right to choose health. For you the payoff will come when you've created a similar discipline in your life. You'll learn what works for you, and what doesn't, what veggies you love and what breads to buy. All of this learning will lead you to your goal—getting into the best shape of your life!

LIVE AND EAT NOW ...
HOW YOU WILL LIVE AND EAT
AT YOUR HEALTHIEST WEIGHT

A good rule of thumb is to eat the amount of calories that a person of your desired body weight consumes. For example: If you weigh 200 lbs. and you'd like to shed about seventy pounds, then you should be consuming the amount of calories of a woman who is 130 pounds. Adopt the behaviors of your desired BMR—Basal Metabolic Rate.

CURRENT BODY	DESIRED BODY
Gender: female	Gender: female
Height: 5'5"	Height: 5'5"
Body: 200 pounds	Target Body: 130 pounds
Daily calories: 2200 per day	Target Calories: 1500 per day

Every week the woman in the example will shed approximately 1.4 pounds; a very healthy amount according to nutritionists, dieticians and physicians. The calorie deficit of 4900 calories per week allows this woman to get healthy in a healthy manner. In a year's time, she will lose the seventy pounds, and will do it by learning new behaviors, creating a positive mental attitude, and she'll have earned the gift of sustained lifestyle skills. Now this is not an exact science but is a guideline. Results will vary depending on your own metabolism and any health or hormone challenges.

Remember in the beginning of the book, I stated that everything can change when you change your thinking? Consider thinking in mileage. This is a fun mind-shift! Statistics show that the average person generally burns 100 calories per mile, walked or run. During our weekly Mind Body F.I.T. community coaching calls, I've heard ladies say things like, "That 500 calorie cupcake was so not worth having to walk 5 miles to burn it off." To start, monitor your calorie consumption, and how many calories you're burning during exercise. This practice will help you create awareness and cause a mindset shift to occur. Don't monitor calorie burns to obsess over it. No! Instead, do it for the perspective shift. Ask yourself, Is it worth it?

Is the chicken cheese quesadilla that is 495 calories worth walking or running 4.95 miles just to break even? My guess is that you will say, "No." If you choose to repeatedly indulge in a high calorie food knowing that your plan is to exercise it off later, you really don't have a very solid plan.

The idea of creating a daily exercise routine is to:

- Create endorphins—endorphins make you feel good

- Get in better shape—increase your fitness level, rev up your metabolism

- Let go of stress—exercise is amazing for your mental health and clarity

- Burn up fat and use it as fuel

If you're constantly eating as many calories as you are burning, then you are simply spinning your wheels. It would be comparable to walking on a treadmill as a way to get to the park. You're not really going anywhere, just staying in place! Empower yourself with this thought: be proactive by learning good nutrition and making better choices. Then the time you spend moving your body will be quality time. Your walk to the park will actually get you there, and it will all be worth your effort.

Does this mean that your entire life should be consumed with calorie counting? Absolutely not. Creating a F.I.T.

and healthy lifestyle is about optimally balancing your life in all areas. Once you have successfully created a lifestyle of health, it will be easy and your decision-making process will be a natural process.

THE GESTATION PERIOD

Have you ever said, "The scale doesn't show my hard work as fast as I want it to; it bums me out so much that I just give in and sabotage myself." Your focus and mindful eating absolutely will show up on the scale. Have a positive expectation of 0.5-2 pounds per week of body shed. This should be your goal. Following this healthy guideline will enable you to shed weight easily while learning over time the skills and mindsets necessary for maintaining. As you've learned throughout this book, there are underlying reasons for an overweight body. Don't miss the learning opportunity of a GO Moment just because you think you're not progressing fast enough. Think of this process as your gestation period to birthing the New You.

It is imperative that you keep in mind the science behind your body chemistry. Remember, 3,500 calories is the equivalent of one pound of body weight. If you get on the scale one day with no change to your body, then weigh the next day to find you are three pounds heavier, don't start tripp'n sista! In order for you to have actually gained three pounds of body weight means that you would have had to consume 10,500 calories since the last time you weighed. That is nearly impossible! Those three pounds could be representation of your body holding water weight. Perhaps you consumed a salty food the day before? Or, just drinking your daily consumption of water intake is equivalent to four pounds. Keep the weighing to a minimum for a truthful reading, and don't let a number on the scale determine your attitude for the day. That is of course ... unless the number is to your liking. Then by all means, celebrate!

What about late night eating? It is a farce that eating late at night will cause weight gain. To be specific, it will only cause weight gain if you have already reached your maximum caloric intake for the day. For instance, let's say your target BMR (amount for losing weight) is 1500 calories per day. If you have already reached your quota at dinner time, and you then decide to eat a 300 calorie snack before bedtime, yes, you will be over your calorie burning quota and you'll gain weight (or not lose weight) on the scale that week. Truth is, when you are eating late, most often it's unnecessary snacking. It's okay to go to bed a little hungry. Why? Because its time to sleep not eat.

What about Intermittent Fasting? Intermittent fasting is another food timing protocol. It does not focus on what you eat, but rather when you eat it. Like any way of eating that proves results, it can become very popularized. Fasting is so tried and true, it goes all the way back to the Bible. I'm not shouting the praises for fasting nor suggesting you fully jump in, but I do want you to consider the importance of a simple rule that qualifies as fasting. Allowing your body a considerable period of time to rest from food digestion is a healthy practice. For instance, having your last meal of the day be dinner and not eating again until breakfast should be normal.

In the next chapter, I'm going to continue our theme of keeping it real. We'll be discussing accountability and showing up in your life. You'll have the opportunity to learn how to begin living as the person you know you can be by gathering all the information and insights you've learned throughout this book and then holding yourself to a new standard. It's exciting to see how much progress you've already made. Let's continue. Say it with me, "I am learning to eat for energy and health."

Chapter 12

The Daily Decision to Show Up

The pain of discipline is far less than the pain of regret.
~ Sarah Bombell

Reaching your healthy lifestyle goals will require adding character to your healthy weight plan. Amongst the most important character traits are discipline, accountability or personal responsibility, and commitment. The many diets you've been on in the past were focused on holding strong with your willpower and exercising your booty off to reach a goal. Well, no more! You can't afford to spend another waking moment worrying about your weight and getting caught up in short-term dieting.

THIS IS ABOUT YOUR LIFE!

You're going to have to reach farther and dig deeper to come into the light of freedom so that you can **Mind-Body Focus**—for good! You say you want to get healthy. Prepare yourself, your character will be tested along this journey. Take a deep breath and settle in. This might take a year or so. Be assured, anything that is to be sustained requires character. Focus on the big picture of what you want for your life and trust yourself that this is the right time to raise your standards.

It's never too late. I once met up with an 83-year-old woman jogging along in a half marathon. I couldn't help but chat with her for a moment; I wanted to know where her drive comes from. She said she's run 150 marathons, and she doesn't even count the half marathons. A widow of ten years, she spends her time training and traveling around the country participating in events. Her grandkids support her by cheering at the finish lines and admiring her wall of medals. She has been interviewed by the news media dozens of times. She says that entering an event keeps her in the mindset of wanting to beat her own time. The kind of drive that Grandma Runner has is a derivative of true character. It's within you as well. You may be using your strength of character in another area of your life and haven't directed it toward your health. Or perhaps it's waiting to be unearthed.

Accountability is about following through and doing what you say you're going to do. As a child you did your chores, which showed personal responsibility and you were rewarded. Perhaps you were rewarded with a weekly allowance, or an "Atta Girl". Now that you're an adult, you can think of creating healthy habits as the chores that must be completed to reach your weekly goal. Your compensation will be your one or two pounds of weight shed at the end of the week or the shift in energy you feel. Some of the ladies in my program also give themselves tangible prizes for reaching their goals. At a five pound mark, they buy a new fitness outfit, or a cool heart rate monitor to celebrate. It's important you discover new ways to celebrate your commitment.

What if being accountable is one of your downfalls? You say you're going to walk three times this week, but you just can't seem to keep to your schedule. You say you're NOT going to sabotage yourself, but you do. Now before you get too down on yourself, rest easy by knowing that many of us have stumbled with truly sticking to a healthy diet. Here's some hope—accountability is a learned behavior. Character is not born into you, it is developed.

For many years I had a lack of personal responsibility. I was relatively unmotivated most of my growing up years. My childhood did not consist of regular chores or responsibilities. In fact, I was not held accountable for much. There was a perceived expectation in my household, but not much follow through in enforcing it. Mom felt detached. She did a lot of talking, but not a lot of connecting. Not being held accountable had an immense effect on my character. My lack of accountability was a factor that contributed to low self-esteem, poor body image and yo-yoing on the scale. But wait a minute, before you think that I am putting the blame on Mom, I would like you to know that I now 'own' the responsibility.

At about the age of 30, I started to put more focus on working on myself. I finally realized that my inability to be accountable greatly affected my body. I had no problem heaving down three bowls of Lucky Charms while alone in the kitchen late at night. I'm sure you've done it. You know, where you pour in a little more milk with your cereal, and then you have too much milk so you add more cereal. Before you know it, you're stomach is stuffed full and you consumed 800 calories. Eating like that is NOT about hunger. Call it boredom, sadness, stress, whatever emotional label you want to put on it, but it's NOT about hunger.

It funneled down to personal accountability. I couldn't fix the emotional eating if I wasn't willing to be responsible for it. It took maturity, soul searching and a handful of hypnotherapy sessions to realize, I am responsible for my own mind and how I choose to use it. Writing this book is my way of shortening the learning curve for you. I figured if I'm extremely frank with you and give you some insights that you have not thought of before, you will be way ahead of the game.

If a behavior is not aligning with how you desire to live your life, then it is your responsibility to do the work to change it. It can be challenging; that's where your courage will come in handy. I am not saying it will be easy, but I am stating that once you take full accountability and own your strengths and weaknesses, you will find it "easier" and feel an incredible source of personal freedom. This is what *"showing up to your life"* means.

Learning to be accountable to yourself with food is about making the right choice when there is no one watching. A girlfriend or a support group is a must-have while on the weight release journey. But true accountability, the kind you will own once you've mastered the inside out approach to weight loss, is a trait you must develop for successful, long-term weight loss and maintenance.

Learn to be okay with putting yourself in check. I often say, "I'm not afraid to call myself out." I encourage you to develop an awareness and honesty within yourself. When you know you've altered from your plan, have the courage to own the mistake. You can't blame it on the circumstances. Like, "Oh I was at a party and everyone was eating cheesecake, so I couldn't help myself." I'll have to call you out on that my friend. If you hear yourself making up an excuse, take personal responsibility. You cannot grow beyond your weakness if you are unwilling to own the stumble. And by the way, its totally okay to eat the damn cheesecake with your girlfriends if you want to, just don't say one thing and do another. That will cause you to distrust yourself.

It's easy to say you are going to do something, and then NOT do it. Or worse, make a promise to yourself, and then NOT follow through to the end result. Perhaps you have thought, *Well, If I haven't said it out loud, no one has to know.* You can indulge in the pie after dinner, and no one will know the difference. It's an easy out, right? Here's the catch: YOUR subconscious is paying attention. Your insides (your hard drive—your unconscious mind and spirit) know better. Your inner computer is keeping track of all the times you didn't follow through. Your subconscious is gathering the information and collectively creating behaviors and systems with that information. Don't think for a minute that you are getting away with not being accountable. It's all being archived.

The habits you have now regarding food, self-esteem and follow through were created from old, stored information derived from your past experiences. If you continue to add to that negative collection of data, you are simply adding to the case against you. The letdown of not being accountable to yourself will trickle through many areas of your life, and it will especially show up on your body through your body. You are the most important person to be accountable to; because when you believe yourself you can live happy knowing you are trustworthy, dependable and show commitment. Having these gifts within your soul allows you to be a better friend and mother, happier spouse, a trusted confidant, respected employer or employee, and most importantly, a person that can MAINTAIN A HEALTHY LIFESTYLE.

To help you in this process, extend your reach. As suggested in Feeling the Fear, connect with girlfriends and teachers, lecturers and trainers! Create a group of women around you that you can answer to with integrity. Because you have respect for them, it is natural to want to please them, therefore you will follow through, take action, and do what you don't like doing, all because you know you want to maintain your integrity with that person. Meaning, when you want to sleep in, but you know your friend is waiting for you at the park to run, you'll get your butt out of bed. This is the easiest way to support your accountability from the outside. You can find formal groups like the Mind Body F.I.T. Community, create your own with your circle of friends, or both.

There are a 2 RULES that will be helpful in order to truly setup a great accountability group.

Rule 1: The group must be comprised of people you admire and respect.

Rule 2: They must be people that you view as successful in the area you want to achieve.

A group I once belonged to offers valuable mentor services to women in business. When you sign up for a one-on-one session with an expert in their field or you sign up to attend a workshop, it is required that you write down your credit card information on the sign up form. When you show up on time and attend the scheduled meeting, your card is not charged for the services. The service you receive, often upwards of $300 a session, is paid for by a funding source and is offered to you as assistance in helping you to achieve your business goals. Now that's a fantastic opportunity, right? But, if you are late or do not attend the scheduled meeting you signed up for, your card is automatically charged a pre-stated nominal fee. This protocol is a phenomenal method for helping women in business to be accountable to their growth process.

Imagine if a friend or mentor laid out 10,000 one dollar bills on your kitchen counter. $10,000. With the money in front of you, she says, "If you stay on track with eating foods that are healthy for you, work hard to create an awareness about why you've been eating for the wrong reasons, exercise your body regularly, and find three ways to be more kind to yourself, you will get to keep this $10,000 at the end of the month." Would you be able to follow through? I'm guessing you said, "Yes, I Can Do It!" If you can do it for $10,000, you can do it without $10,000. Do it for you!

Creating a successful accountability system is key to the process. Use both external and internal resources to help you create permanent behaviors. At first it may be challenging, but soon you'll find it's the new way you live. First you'll recognize the GO Moments (Growth Opportunity), then you'll reach the next level. You'll be able to choose "YOU over food".

Check out the 4 Stages of Learning as an example to the progress you seek.

Accountability-Applying the 4 Stages of Learning

This example is based on the 4 Stages of Competence established in 1963 by Paul Curtis and Phillip Warren.

Stage 1 – Unconscious Incompetence

I ate the cookie, then two more, then went back for one more.

Stage 2 – Conscious Incompetence

I ate the cookie, felt guilty, but it was so good I didn't care. I knew while I was eating it that I shouldn't be.

Stage 3 – Conscious Competence

As I was eating the cookie, I realized I was eating the cookie. I asked myself, "Why am I really eating the cookie?" I took a bite of the cookie and said to myself, "The cookie is good, but I am BETTER."

Stage 4 – Unconscious Competence

I love my body, and myself. Sometimes I eat one, sometimes I don't. I've learned to manage emotions in other healthy ways.

KEY DRIVERS

It is important to begin to understand what motivates you to be healthier? What lights you up? We all have very individual motivating factors. What are yours? If you want to get in the best shape of your life, you're going to have to discover your Key Drivers, and employ them. Dig deep my friend.

What motivates you to get out of bed in the morning?

_____

_____

_____

What turns you on in life?

_____

_____

_____

What keeps you awake at night and gets you excited?

_____

_____

_____

What experiences have you unexpectedly encountered that resonate with you?

_____

_____

_____

If you don't have the quick answer to those questions, then its time you do some soul searching. With a little mindful ingenuity, and an honest look in the mirror, I bet you could find a way to connect shedding weight with discovering a new passion.

As I shared with you earlier, when I started running, I didn't expect it to be a life-changing experience. I just figured it would be a great way to stay in shape and connect with my super hero sister-in-law. Yet it unexpectedly provided me great reward. The discipline of running enabled me to overcome self-limiting beliefs, taught me how to achieve goals and provided me valuable personal development insight that I could then pass on to you.

It doesn't have to be running—although I do encourage you to give it a go. It is the single most natural and innate exercise your body knows, and you can do it anywhere. Perhaps you can turn a hobby, interest or life struggle into a passion. You could help others by reaching out and offering a hand up. By stepping out of your comfort zone and doing an activity that you've never done before, you may find that you get so lit up with excitement that it becomes a driving force in your life. The character you learn can transfer to your weight loss journey and help you succeed. It will fill you up in a way that food cannot.

You could sign up for a run/walk that raises money for a cause you want to support. The Susan G. Komen Foundation Race for the Cure started with a 5K walk in 1983 involving 800 participants. Because of the determination to make her sister's life count, Nancy Brinker, founder of Susan G. Komen Foundation, spearheaded a global movement involving over a million race participants and reportedly raising over one billion dollars. I would bet that Nancy Brinker had no idea that she was capable of creating such a force when she started. Imagine the spirit-filled emotion she must carry in her heart knowing she's made a difference.

The idea here is to take a potential passion, and build from it. Like building a house made of bricks. You don't start on the second story; you begin at the foundation and place one brick at a time. But you do have to start! Mark Victor Hanson says, "Don't wait until everything is just right. It will never be perfect. There will always be challenges, obstacles and less than perfect conditions. So what. Get started now. With each step you take, you will grow stronger, and stronger, more and more skilled, more and more self-confident, and more and more successful."

Even if you are the most unmotivated person in the world, I know that there are things in your life that mean something to you. I am asking you to tap into that meaning, and use it as a catalyst to become more optimistic, love your life, believe in yourself, and shed the unneccessary weight. If you feel you need motivation to get you started, know that you cannot wait for someone else to give it to you. You must create it! Don't wait for another person to initiate it; it's not as potent that way.

In one marathon, I started to feel my energy dip about halfway through. I thought to myself, *Okay De'Anna, you gotta kick it up a notch.* But I wasn't quite sure how to do that. I recalled that a good friend with a lot of marathon experience advised me to derive energy from the cheering onlookers as I pass by them. So my plan was to soak in their yelling and cheering as I ran by.

At one of the most crowded turns in the course, I noticed that people on the sidelines were just standing there with their homemade signs. They weren't yelling, nor screaming like I needed from them. They were probably saving it up for their family member or friend, but I didn't care what the reason, I needed their energy. So in an effort to spark up some motivation, I decided to take on the responsibility and yell at them! Yes, I know, it's a backwards approach, but I was dragging and I needed to do something about it. I screamed, "Come on, give it up for your runners, make some noise!"

As soon as the words screeched from my single voice, I received hundreds of yells back at me. Just thinking about it now as I write, makes the hairs on my neck stand on end. It was an emotionally moving moment. They cheered loudly, smiled wide, and pumped their fists! I learned something that day, and began to use it as my strategy thereafter. It's a tactic that is useful not only for marathons, but for life. The message I received was: *You must be the spark that generates the fire.*

Your one small gesture will ricochet tenfold, and you'll receive enough motivation to accomplish anything you can dream up! If you want to let weight go, and never regain it, it's important that you take the lead, and *design the life you desire.* Your contagious spirit will be a never-ending state of perpetual energy.

YOUR INTERNAL COMMITMENT

As you've now discovered, this methodology involves your mind, your body and your spirit. I believe you can only get healthy and stay that way when you involve your whole self. It's vital that you stop trying to compartmentalize your life.

Imagine with this approach how your journey can be different from this point on. Every time I enter a race event, whether it's with the Mind Body F.I.T. ladies or on my own, I move amongst the thousands of people in attendance thinking, they showed up to their lives today. We could have all slept in, but we didn't, we showed up to enjoy our health.

In the end, it's not about the food. It's not about the weight. It's about showing up to your best life. As you utilize the mindsets and insights provided in this book, you'll become trained and skilled at knowing how to navigate yourself. Before long you will have crossed the threshold from in training to maintaining a fit life.

Your age does not matter. As 104 year old running world record holder, Ida Keeling says "My secret is in my head. Don't sit around doin' nothin. Get up and do somethin'. See how different you feel."

Make the internal commitment to yourself now.

"I now commit to my best life."

Signed:

JAYLENE'S STORY

Jaylene, an inspiring Mind Body F.I.T. Club member, has shed 105 pounds. She has achieved such impressive results by following the guidelines I have shared with you in these pages. She was obese for all of her adult life and is now enjoying a body that can move easily, run up hills and fit into skinny jeans. She is more than thrilled to fit into a size that she never has before, but what is truly soulful is her overwhelming feeling of accomplishment.

Facing a lifetime of buried emotions, Jaylene took on a courageous journey to revealing the hidden sadness she stored inside. For many years, she went on about her life raising children, being a good wife and submerging the abuse she had suffered as a child. When she joined the program, she had already endured a midlife breakdown, and was seeking counseling to help her put the pieces of her life back together. Our program resonated with her, like sunlight breaking through the clouds.

Through MBFC *Daily Soul Question and Subconscious Integration* tools, Jaylene discovered that she allowed people to control her most of her life. She also learned that she had feelings of not being good enough. On a coaching call one evening she said, "I decided that I'm not going to just eat it anymore." All of us on the call knew that she meant, she could stand up for herself and have a voice. Not only was it incredible to hear her own her power, but it was also very revealing. Through her own words, "Not going to eat it anymore," she unknowingly exposed the root to her obesity struggles.

Amazing, isn't it? Our minds are so powerful. She had been 'eating it' for years.

Jaylene has blossomed as we've watched her shed her old shell. Her talents and abilities have shown up full force. She's now attracting a new sense of happiness, purpose and more prosperity in her life. People she comes in contact with are inspired by her. The barista at Starbucks, the dressing room attendant, the women jogging next to us in a race; everyone wants what she's got! As her coach, when I think about her journey, I can attribute her success to one thing. And that is *Showing Up*. She shows up to her life every day by instilling her character.

She believed herself to be too uncoordinated to run. We even heard her say, "I can't run." But she recognized her self-limiting belief and started practicing discipline. She did learn to run and is now participating in triathlons and half marathons. She also rides her bike often exploring longer miles and new territory. Jaylene has shown up by doing the 'right' things on a daily basis; eating for energy, in the right amount, moving her body, embracing her spirit, loving herself more and then just simply repeating those behaviors daily.

Repeat ... repeat ... repeat ... each day. One day of success, repeated until it became a week of success. She lost one pound consistently each week, and celebrates that one pound like it is twenty pounds. One week turned into a month, and a month has turned into a year. She's now 105 pounds leaner and has completely earned her new body.

L ife can feel stressful on some days. To live at your greatest health and happiness, it takes a commitment to your own growth and resilience to continually overcome. In transitional times especially, we've got to stay focused on what we want, rather than don't want. It's so easy to get off track.

How do we stay focused? More consistent?

The key is to be in a progress mindset. Keep learning self-awareness, develop more real confidence and give daily effort knowing it doesn't have to be stressful or time-consuming. As an advocate for personal leadership, I encourage you to keep stretching what you believe you can do. Grandma was an example to vital health; jogging into her late 90s and smiling with every step. I am willing to carry that baton and be the example for you. You can do this, especially when you have support like I am offering.

We are rolling out more online courses, fun and in-depth workshops and opportunities to coach with me one on one. Why? Because these are my growth goals, too. I've made it my purpose to shine a light within and help others do the same. Growing up in a dysfunctional environment, I know the self-growth it took me to finally mature and claim a better life. I went from the rebellious chick smoking under the bleachers in high school, voting myself least likely to succeed to a confident woman speaking to thousands and becoming an adult athlete. I learned to grow and rise above. Advancing your personal development and upholding physical self-care is the foundation to all other success in your life. Rise like you've never risen before.

About the Author

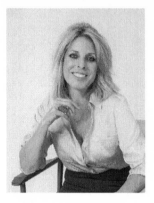

As a teenager, De'Anna Nunez battled with body-shaming, low self-worth, self abuse, drug use and eating disorders. When she became a mom at twenty, she knew she wanted more for her life, so she set out on a s-hero's journey to discover that possibility.

De'Anna earned an initial education in Clinical Hypnotherapy and rocked the stage for more than two decades performing more than a 1,000+ Hypnosis presentations to over 500,000 live audience members. She became one of an elite group of women that have successfully presented Hypnosis in a multitude of industries including television, radio, corporate, military, theme parks, education (high schools and colleges), large public fairs and festivals.

She's since continued her education in Hypnosis instructor training, mental performance, Humanistic Neuro-Linguistic Psychology, advanced personal development coaching, sports nutrition, run coaching and group fitness.

As a personal achievement, she has a decade of experience running over 100 marathon distances where she learned and practiced the power of mindset, belief and responsible nutrition.

Her clients are now diverse – from executives, entrepreneurs and athletes to everyday people who have a desire to overcome self-limited thinking. Her purpose is to empower people. Like Yoda to Luke Skywalker, you and De'Anna become a trusted team. She gets in your head and makes you a believer too. Whether you ever run a single step, her teachings will surely impact your life as she shares success is not a secret, it's a system.

MIND BODY FIT CLUB

The Mind Body Fit Club is an online, interactive community where you can implement and habitize De'Anna's teachings alongside inspiring women from across the U.S., Canada and soon the world.

It's fun, uplifting and life changing!

Her F.I.T. Method – Focus, Inward, and Target can strategically...

- Reveal and Release subconscious mental blocks
- Reframe your confidence in your mind and body
- Break through outdated beliefs about who you are
- Transform emotional and stress eating
- Abolish Sugar Cravings
- Reboot Mindset, Metabolism and Energy
- Enjoy your life from a 100% Anti-Diet approach
- Release Extra Weight

Go to **MindBodyFitClub.com** to enroll in the *Change Up Your Life Challenge* Now!

(Use code **MBFC** for **$100 savings**)

WORK *with*
DE'ANNA
Nunez

De'Anna Nunez is a dynamic Keynote Speaker and is available to speak to your company or organization. She also offers private coaching and a weekly group-Coaching membership. All Top-Achievers have a mindset Coach and so should you!
Go to DeAnnaNunez.com

**Connect with De'Anna
on Social Media!**

LinkedIn: @DeAnnaNunez
Twitter: @DeAnnaNunez
Instragram: @DeAnnaJNunez
Facebook: @DeAnnaJNunez
Facebook.com/mindbodyfitclub

Made in the USA
Middletown, DE
03 October 2020